How to Deal Simply
with
Back Pain
and
Rheumatoid Joint Pain

A Preventive and Self-Treatment Manual
For Those Who Prefer to Adhere to the
Logic of the Natural and the Simple

By

F. Batmanghelidj

Global Health Solutions, Inc.
Back Pain
P.O. Box 3189
Falls Church, VA 22043 USA

ISBN 0-9629942-0-0

Book design: Xanthus Design 202/408-1898

The use of photographs from the anatomical models has been made possible
by kind permission of the Anatomical Chart Company of Chicago.

*I thank God for having given me the ability
to make this presentation.*

*This book is dedicated to those who
have suffered from severe pain,
low back or otherwise,
and have experienced its devastating impact;
of these people,
to my friend, James H.G., in particular.*

*To the late
Mr. Arthur Dickson-Wright
the last of the great general surgeons, a wit
and a humanitarian pioneer in cancer research.*

Also, to my family.

Disclaimer

The information and exercises presented in this book are based on the training, personal experience, and extensive research of the author. The author of this book does not dispense medical advice or prescribe the use of any technique as a form of treatment for physical or medical problems without the advice of a physician, either directly or indirectly. The intent of the author is only to offer information of a general nature based on the knowledge of anatomy and the science of physiology to help prevent future back and rheumatoid joint problems. This book is not intended as a replacement for sound medical advice from a physician. Application of the concepts, procedures and exercises described herein are undertaken at the individual's own risk. The procedures depicted should be undertaken in strict compliance with instructions given herein. Pregnant women, previously injured persons, and individuals with prior back injuries or who have any other pre-existing pathological or orthopedic condition or injury should not undertake procedures contained in this booklet without prior consultation with a qualified physician.

All recommendations and exercises herein contained are made without guarantees on the part of the author or the publisher, their agents, or employees. The author and publisher disclaim all liability in connection with the use of the information presented herein.

Contents

Chapter 5

About the Author

Dr. F. Batmanghelidj ("Batman-ge-lij"—who did not wish to be licensed for "practice of pharmaceutically oriented and invasive medicine in the U.S.") received formal medical training at St. Mary's Hospital Medical School (London University). His research into the phenomenon of pain and water metabolism of the body has dictated a *paradigm change* in the basic understanding of science applied to the practice of medicine. His views are published in scientific journals. The underlying principles of the recommendations in his treatment procedures are the most current knowledge of anatomy and the science of physiology.

Since a highly significant and basic paradigm change in the practice of medicine, in the face of very stiff commercial and professional resistance, will be difficult to institute unless there is a concurrent public educational program to force the change, it has become necessary to begin a highly coordinated public awareness program. The author believes: *"To end major diseases on earth within two decades is now a possibility. A paradigm change in the science of medicine will do it, but the public must demand the change. The time to act is now."*

For production of educational materials for the public, under legal advisement, it became necessary to establish *Global Health Solutions Inc.*, a legally independent enterprise. This self-treatment manual, *How to Deal Simply with Back Pain and Rheumatoid Joint Pain*, and the videotape *How to Deal with Back Pain* are the first of these educational products.

Preface:
The Foundation for the Simple
in Medicine

In 1983, the Foundation for the Simple in Medicine, a charitable medical research (think tank) foundation, was founded to establish grounds for a change in the present fundamental understanding of the basis on which all human applied research has been done. The present basic assumption in practice of medicine (paradigm) is that it is the physico-chemical properties of ions (*"i-ons"* are the purest form of the basic elements, such as sodium, potassium, calcium, magnesium, etc.) that regulate the water intake of the body, and that the substance we call "water," the solvent of the body, performs a passive role to these basic elements and everything else that is dissolved in the same solvent.

Why? Because early in research, it was recognized that *solutes* (substances that are dissolved in the body fluids) are highly reactive substances. Clinical experience (articles 23, 24, 25, 26, 2, 3, 6, 9 in the bibliography at the end of the book) has shown that this assumption can not be complete, because the body can become dehydrated as we progress in age. The Foundation holds the opinion that since the sensor regulators to ion exchanges that regulate the water movement in the body are proteins, and proteins by nature are obedient in the presence of water, the more free water there is around them, the more efficiently these proteins function.[38] It therefore follows that it must be water that ultimately regulates its own intake.

Clinically, this view can be validated by the fact that people who do not acknowledge thirst even though dehydrated, after a few days of regulating their water intake on a "forced voluntary" basis, will rediscover their thirst sensation—their body's craving for water. The Foundation is making another statement which follows the logic of the previous view: Since all functions of the body are water-dependent, let us revise our approach to medical treatment procedures; let us recognize a primary water regulatory role for the neurotransmitter systems that have been recognized to be involved in the water intake mechanisms of the body. In the medical conditions where these systems are being chemically manipulated to make the patient "better," let us try to satisfy the natural urge of these systems for water *before* there is any chemical interference with their systems' other natural emergency regulatory functions. The systems recognized for water regulation of the body are: *serotonergic* (regulates the calcium movement of the cell, and pain registration among many other functions), *histaminergic* (regulates cat-i-ons—cations are the basic elements that carry a positive electric charge—exchange in the cell, also recognized in many other functions, induction of pain and allergy) and *renin-angiotensin* (stimulated into activity by the two previous systems independently and possibly simultaneously, manipulated in hypertension).

To introduce its ideas into the practice of medicine all over the world, the Foundation has begun the publication of its scientific views in its own *Science in Medicine Simplified* (Sci. Med. Simplified), which is periodically printed and distributed to research centers and medical libraries in different parts of the world.

Invitation to Readers

Let us lobby together and ask the scientists in medicine to begin the evaluation of the statements dictated by the new paradigm that recognizes the regulatory and reactive hydrolytic functions of water in the body.[6] Under the new paradigm, you can rest assured, the practice of medicine will become a much gentler *preventive*, as well as curative, physiological approach to early disease emergence, *before* the damage is done.

We are most interested in hearing your reactions to this book, and about success or relief you may achieve by following the suggestions and exercises presented herein.

If you follow the program and recommendations and do not experience relief, we would like to hear about that as well. The comments of physicians and other health-care professionals will be particularly appreciated.

Please send comments, reactions, and suggestions to:

Back Pain
P.O. Box 3189
Falls Church, Virginia 22043 USA

All responses will be held in strictest confidence.

Introduction

Back Pain, Disc Displacement, Rheumatoid Joint Pain: Water and Exercise

This educational preventive-treatment manual will deal with chronic back and rheumatoid joint pain in language as simple as possible, although the impact of what is being said will eventually fill volumes of written material. The reader is advised not to judge the value of this book by its simplicity of presentation, but should try to evaluate the essence of what is being said. Justification of confused views will always produce voluminous verbiage, particularly when held views have to have an application appeal for the people who are at the receiving end, and if it eventually will mean expensive surgical interferences.

If we are to prevent decompensation and/or achieve relief from pain of disc dispacement, we have to make sure that our body is optimally hydrated so that water can leave the main circulatory systems and hydrate the disc core; also, that the front angle of the intervertebral spaces is kept widely open, until corrective restitution to the physical properties and position of the disc have taken place: How do we do this?

You are encouraged to read this book in its entirety; however, a preliminary reading of the first part of the manual will clearly illuminate how it is possible to alleviate the pain and anxiety of back discomfort, mild or excruciating. The more detailed part of the manual should then be read to revise and learn more about the physiology of pain, the cell, the nerves sensitive to pain; referred pain and/or muscle weakness caused by a prolapsed intervertebral disc; weight and motion and their effect; the foot and its arches; special points about pelvic anatomy and distribution of forces; the relationship of the disc to the vertebra; the disc and its functions; and the cartilage and the joints.

Simple exercises and hydrolic treatment (regulated water intake) are carefully explained.

Here, then, is a guide to the care and preventive treatment of back pain and disc displacement, as well as rheumatoid joint pain.

Chapter 1
Chronic Pain: What Does It Signify?

This book started as a simple address of back pain, which, as everyone knows, is a devastating chronic pain of the human body. As my research at the Foundation into the phenomemon of pain has steadily progressed, I realized that this book would be incomplete if some explanation on the "other" chronic joint pain of the body—rheumatoid arthritis—was not included. After all, most back pain originates at the vertebral joints, and if this book was to be a grass-roots approach to pain, rheumatoid joint pain is an equally devastating condition that also deserved discussion. The fundamental explanations about the origin of rheumatoid joint pain are equally simple, and, at the outset, it is even more simply treatable than back pain.

A news item in the 31 July 1990 Health section of *The Washington Post* gave me sufficient emotional shock to restructure this book, which was at that time already in the printer's hands.

A 47-year-old child psychiatrist had been suffering from severe rheumatoid arthritis for some time. She had been given the customary medications until she had developed addiction, apparently, and the combination of addiction and pain had totally incapacitated her. She had a daughter of 17, who was brain-damaged and asthmatic, and a son who was bright. The stress in the family setting had become so great that even the housekeeper suffered a heart attack. The psychiatrist's husband, himself a doctor and a prominent cancer researcher, eventually found the situation unbearable enough that he took the lives of his wife and two children and then committed suicide.

To my mind, this tragedy—along with similar, daily-occurring tragedies—stemmed from a most absurd ignorance and the "ostrich" policy of those involved in the politics of medicine. The scientific knowledge that can offer simple solutions to major health problems—most particularly, at a preventable stage that would not cause severe genetic damage—does exist.

For the innocent and trusting sick to benefit from the solutions offered within the science of physiology, medicine will need a change of stand by some key policy-makers and the government administrators of health who support the present commercial attitude of the health-care industry; medical professionals will need to give support to alternative ideas and the more plausible science-based solutions to the health problems of the sick. This change of attitude might not serve the profit motivations of the industrial and commercial arms of the health-care institutions, but it should be remembered that simple, nature-serving solutions to major health problems are less costly to the society they are *obligated* to serve.

The Cell

Let us take a look at the most basic life-generating element in the body, the cell. The cell is surrounded by a very thin outer "skin" or membrane that protects it from being flooded by unregulated entry of water, salt, sugar, fats, and many other elements that constitute the serum solution that is outside the cell wall.

Since the cell is constantly bathed in serum solution, it regulates its intake and output by means of many, many small *pumping units*. Fluid inside the cells should be neutral, neither too acidic nor too alkaline; it has a pH of 7.4 under normal circumstances.* The way this neutral pH is maintained is very simple: the *cation* (cat-i-on) pumps constantly pump out hydrogen ion, which is the acid substance not used by the cell. The entire body—nerve tissue, bone, cartilage, ligament, muscle, blood, brain, you name it—is made up of these tiny cells, each performing this regulation of intake and output of elements to maintain function. Each cell is just like an underwater city, with canal systems and waterways; outside of it, arteries and veins are its highways.

---

*7.4 is the level of reading on a scale designed to measure the degree of acidity. From 1 to 7 is the acid range; 1 being more acid than 7. From 7 to 14 on the scale is the alkaline range; 7 is less alkaline than 14. On the pH scale, 7 is neutral.

Water and Life

The most important life-giving substance in the body, and one that the body desperately depends on, is *water*. In the soft tissues—muscle, liver, kidney, the intestines—75 percent of the volume of the cells is water. The brain cell is said to be 85 percent water. The first impact of dehydration is felt by the brain cells; they are very sensitive to water loss from the body and their functions would be affected by even minute changes in their water contents. The above figures roughly represent a normal, healthy state of function. The blood and fluids outside the cells consist of approximately 94 percent water.

Water has the urge and determination to flow from solutions at lower concentration to solutions at higher concentration when these solutions are separated by a thin membrane. When the concentration of water is 94 percent outside the cell and 75 percent inside the cell, there is a tendency for water to flow across the cell membrane into the cell. This difference of 19 percent acts somewhat like the waterhead of a hydroelectric dam. Nature has designed a simple mechanism of providing each cell with hydroelectric power. It uses this 19 percent difference in water levels to generate electricity inside the cell. In the same way that the height of water over the turbine generators of a hydroelectric dam turns the generators and creates electricity, at the cell wall barrier, water turns the cation pumps and generates electricity.

Water—The Energy of Life

Energy from the electricity that is generated by the pump units is stored in small energy pool units or "batteries" called *ATP*. From this energy pool the cell draws the necessary power to perform its various functions, such as transmission of information in the nerves, cell growth, cell division, and manufacture and secretion of some final products that the cell is naturally designed to produce. The food we eat mainly provides the raw materials for the wear and tear and some energy for the repair; a smaller portion of energy required for the myriads of functional activities is taken from food. If we drink regularly and enough, the main bulk of energy used by the body is normally and naturally generated from hydro-electric power at the level of the individual cells.

Since all nerve transmissions depend in a major way on the hydroelectric energy of water, insufficient water intake can also cause a chronic fatigue state of the body.

Acidity and the Cell

If for some reason the pumps of a certain region do not work properly, allowing acid to build up in an area, after a certain level of acidity is reached, the chemical reaction converts two of the elements to substances called *kinins*. These kinins and their subordinate products (K agents) are pain producers, indicating that the acidity of the region is increased and that there is not enough "waterhead" to drive the acid-clearing pumps. It's as simple as that!

These kinins have two main natural functions. One is to cause pain to immobilize the area that is short of water when the cells of the region cannot carry out all the water-dependent actions. The other equally important function is to begin a shunting system of circulation to bring more blood and supplies to the region. It should be remembered that water deficiency of the cell means cell damage, particularly when it reaches a pain-producing level. It should also be remembered that although adequate water intake could prevent pain-producing levels of local or general dehydration, when cell damage has taken place, in most cases (and particularly in bone and joint pains), the hasty act of increased water intake cannot reverse the situation immediately. The local damage will be repaired according to a pattern that takes time.

The water content of the body is in two states: *free water* and *bound water*. Bound water is busy with the maintenance of other functions and is not available for new work. Free water, as its name implies, is available to perform other physiological functions, in much the same way that cash flow gets things done. Bound water is like fixed assets; it is credit but not readily dispensable.

To get your body's "cash flow" topped up, you need to work for it and drink water. *Don't wait to get pain.* Drink water on regular basis, even if you are not thirsty. Don't imagine that a dry mouth is the only indication of thirst; *chronic pain also is often an indication of regional thirst, particularly in rheumatoid arthritic joints of the hands, knees, etc.* Some of these points will be discussed separately.

With increase in age, we lose our thirst sensation. We can be thirsty for one glass of water when our body might actually need two, three, or more glasses to be "topped up." *Even a few drops of water can make the difference to an important bodily function.*

The daily routine of the body depends on a turnover of about 40,000 glasses of water. The body recycles this volume of water in 24 hours, but at the end it needs a minimum top-up of about six glasses in twenty-four hours. *Tea, coffee and alcohol are not to be considered as water;* these are *drying* agents, and they force water out of the body. In the summer and humid periods, and during continuous exercise (particularly in the summer) the human body needs more water for its cooling system (perspiration and sweating)— sometimes up to 10 to 15 or even *more* glasses a day.

When you drink this amount of water, you should not maintain a salt-free diet. Otherwise you will develop cramps, because salt is involved in pushing acid out of the cell and from the body. Higher intake of water will mean a greater loss of salt from the body. Water by itself is the best natural diuretic. Increases in daily urine volume will mean a comparative increase in loss of salt from the body, which may produce complications of its own.

Chapter 2
Low Back Pain

Low back pain is a problem of contemporary mankind, particulary in advanced societies. In Europe it is a major health issue. In France it is called the "malady of the century." In America, well over 40 million people suffer from back pain and a large number of them are often confined to bed as a result of severe back pain; back pain results in an $80 billion-a-year health cost to these same people.

A sophisticated "business" approach to this problem of society is ever-expanding. In America alone, well over 200,000 severe cases from this patient group are operated on every year—often for a second, third, or even a fourth time. Perhaps you have suffered already, or maybe you wish to take preventive measures. In either case, this educational presentation can be the breakthrough know-how and technology to the future prevention of the problems associated with chronic joint pains.

The information and the series of scientifically designed exercises are intended to show a natural and simple appproach to the problem. By applying these techniques, you could prevent the progress of the initial low back pain to the more advanced stages of disc degeneration, to the point of requiring drastic manipulative treatment or surgery.

The approach to the understanding of the problems of low back pain explained in this manual applies to those with sciatic pain as well.

The simple chronic low back or rheumatoid joint pains of the hands or knees are initial signals of the body that should be taken very seriously. Normally, pain indicates a need to limit the activity of the region. When pain is felt in the lower back repeatedly and often (chronic pain), in the vast majority of cases, it is an indicator that the hinge section that connects the pressure of weight of the upper body (head, neck, chest, abdomen and its contents) to the pelvis and transfers this weight onto the legs finds this burden too great. The pain is an indicator for either the limitation and decrease of the burden of weight of the upper body mass on the weight-bearing lumbar region (the spinal vertebrae), or the strengthening of the points of transfer of the upper body weight to the pelvis and the legs. The lower back area is the site of weight distribution beween the spine, which supports all the upper body weight, and the pelvis, to which it connects.

Before getting into the relationship of lower back and sciatic pain, you should become aware of some new ideas on the meaning of pain and how it develops. When you learn about the mechanism of pain production, like a master key that fits many locks, you will be able to relate the information to many different kinds of chronic pain, including chronic rheumatoid joint pains that reign terror on many elderly sufferers. The pain indicator has the same meaning between the weight-bearing joints of the spine and the force-enduring activity of the finger joints that grip, move, and carry weights, be they shopping bags or a chair that is moved from one position to another. It is the joint surfaces that endure the impact and pressure of "force" and the muscles that have to contract and relax for the work to be done.

The Brain and the Spinal Column

We all know that the nervous system is made up of the brain and the spinal cord. The brain is housed in the skull and the spinal cord is situated in the length of the spinal column, all the way down to the *sacrum*, or back bone of the pelvis.

The spinal column is made up of 24 vertebrae. The neck region has seven small and very delicate vertebrae, the chest or thorax has 12 gradually thicker and larger vertebrae, and the low back or lumbar region has five even thicker and larger vertebrae. The sacrum (tailbone) is the largest of the vertebrae that is composed from fusion of a few of the lower vertebrae. Also note the curvatures of the spine that allow it to act as a "coiled spring" (a series of disc "springs" under constant tension)—Fig. 1.

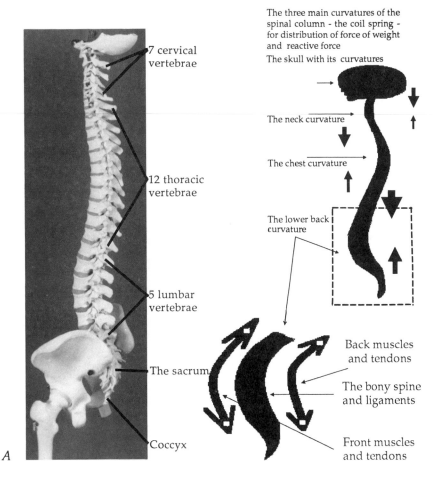

The three main curvatures of the spinal column - the coil spring - for distribution of force of weight and reactive force

The skull with its curvatures

7 cervical vertebrae

The neck curvature

The chest curvature

12 thoracic vertebrae

The lower back curvature

5 lumbar vertebrae

The sacrum

Back muscles and tendons

The bony spine and ligaments

Coccyx

Front muscles and tendons

A

B

Fig. 1: *A-An anatomical model demonstrates the variation in size of each vertebra from neck downward, the natural curvature of the spine, and the position of the discs.*

B-Shows how the natural curvatures are created to give a "coiled spring" property to the whole of the spinal column.

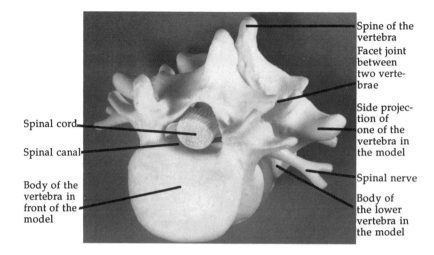

Spine of the vertebra

Facet joint between two verte-brae

Side projec-tion of one of the vertebra in the model

Spinal nerve

Body of the lower vertebra in the model

Spinal cord

Spinal canal

Body of the vertebra in front of the model

Fig. 2: *Front and side views of a model of two adjoining vertebrae showing the position of the spinal cord in the spinal canal, the nerve leaving the foramen, and the position of one of the facet joints between the two vertebrae.*

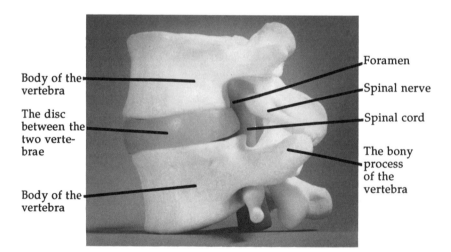

Foramen

Spinal nerve

Spinal cord

The bony process of the vertebra

Body of the vertebra

The disc between the two verte-brae

Body of the vertebra

Fig. 3: *Model of two vertebrae, showing the position of the disc, the spinal cord, the spinal nerve and the foramen, where the spinal nerve leaves the spinal canal.*

As you can see, each vertebra has a body, two side projec-tions, and a back projection called a spine. There is a hollow space between the body and the spinal projection of each of the vertebrae. The bone structures around the hollow spaces of the adjoining vertebrae are joined together from above and below by the attachment of ligaments and fibrous bands. As a result of the serial connection of these hollow spaces, a long canal system is formed, which runs the length of the spinal column from the connection of the neck and the skull to the sacrum. Through this canal run the spinal cord and the nerves that come out and go to the muscles and the skin. These nerves also provide the ability to sense touch, heat, and pain—Fig. 2.

The different parts of these bone structures are connected to their counterparts above and below by ligaments and tendons—Figs. 3 and 4.

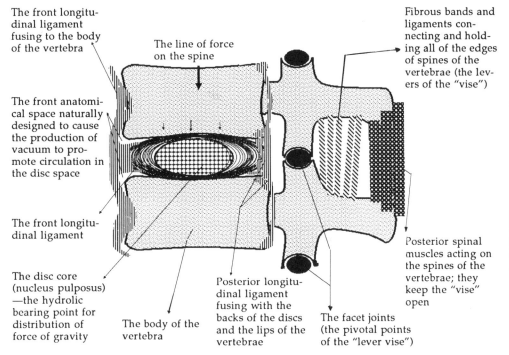

The front longitudinal ligament fusing to the body of the vertebra

The line of force on the spine

Fibrous bands and ligaments connecting and holding all of the edges of spines of the vertebrae (the levers of the "vise")

The front anatomical space naturally designed to cause the production of vacuum to promote circulation in the disc space

The front longitudinal ligament

The disc core (nucleus pulposus)—the hydrolic bearing point for distribution of force of gravity

The body of the vertebra

Posterior longitudinal ligament fusing with the backs of the discs and the lips of the vertebrae

The facet joints (the pivotal points of the "lever vise")

Posterior spinal muscles acting on the spines of the vertebrae; they keep the "vise" open

Fig 4: *The two vertebrae keep the disc in position as if they were the two faces of a vise—the hydrolic force of the disc core prevents the "vise" from closing. The whole problem of disc degeneration will begin by the initial decrease of the hydrolic force of the disc core.*

The Disc

Lodged between these 24 vertebrae are positioned 23 soft, joint-packing discs. These discs are the spinal column's spacings and shock absorbers, as well as the roller bearings that allow one vertebra to regulate position *vis-a-vis* the vertebrae above and below—Fig. 1.

A fundamental law of physics states that for every action there is an equal and opposite reaction. This law applies to the human body as well. Each time you force your weight on the ground when standing, walking, or running, your feet have to put up with a similar force being transmitted to them from the ground. Each foot nullifies some of that force, but some will travel up the leg and reach the pelvis, where some more of the force is nullified in the pelvic area through the circular nature of the organ. But some force travels up the spine; here the role of the discs is to dampen all that force so that nothing gets up to the brain to cause damage—Figs. 5 and 6.

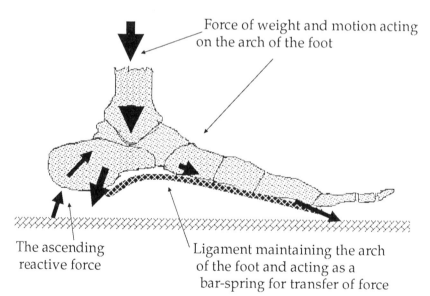

Force of weight and motion acting on the arch of the foot

The ascending reactive force

Ligament maintaining the arch of the foot and acting as a bar-spring for transfer of force

Fig 5: *The foot and the force of weight and the reactive force reflected from the ground.*

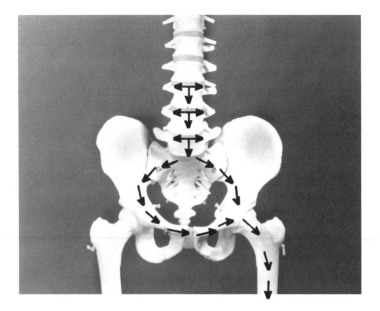

Fig. 6A: *Model of the pelvis and the lumbar vertebrae demonstrating the approximate distribution of the lines of force of weight reaching the ground in the process of walking. These lines of force shift from one leg to the other as steps are taken.*

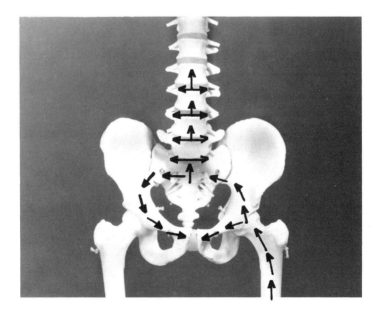

Fig. 6B: *The lines of reactive force moving upward.*

How can a simple disc do so much work? *The disc's water-absorbing properties allow it to perform its nature-allocated functions.* The disc absorbs water, becomes taut, and packs the joint to act as a wedge between the vertebrae, where the muscles of the back and front make the vertebral column a firm anatomical unit, maintaining the normal curvatures that permit the spine to also act as a spring. The center of gravity of the body, even with its well-packed spinal column joints, acts forward of the body—which is why your feet are directed to grow toward the front! The muscles of the back keep pulling on the column all the time to keep the posture upright. When the discs are fully hydrated and firm, they are effective wedges, particularly in the lumbar region, reducing the demand on the back muscles.

Consider this: Over 80 percent of all back pains are caused by muscle spasm.

If the discs are not fully hydrated and their wedge quality is poor, it becomes the increasing responsibility of the back muscles to keep the body upright. More work is done, and since water is required to keep the cation(acid-clearing) pumps going at the same time that this water should have been used to expand the disc, pain is registered in that area. This pain is an indicator of a regional water deficiency that affects the muscles of the back, as well as the discs between the vertebrae that are being squeezed by the pressure of the weight of the upper part of the body.

During the earlier phase of pain-producing spasm of the muscles, treatment with painkillers and even some exercises or manipulations to release the tension can temporarily reduce or even remove the pain. But the basic understanding of how the pain arose is absolutely essential to prevent recurrence of the problem. It should also be remembered that the dehydration that has produced the back pain signal can also be doing damage at other non-pain-registering sites, such as the kidney, the liver, or even the brain cells (which are highly sensitive to even minute levels of water deficiency). If a pregnant woman, before the stage of actual physical burden of pregnancy, has had or develops very early chronic pain of the joints, be they the lower vertebral joints (back pain) or the finger joints, she should consider this pain a sign of her own dehydration, which can seriously affect her child.

During the night, while you sleep, the disc absorbs water from its surroundings, because it has no blood vessels of its own. There must be enough free water in the region for it to be able to rehydrate itself. During the day, when you are upright and moving, the force of your weight in motion (which is *more* than your actual scale weight) will force water out of your discs and into the vertebrae above and below. This release can cause a shrinkage in height of about one and a half to two centimeters during 12 hours. Bed rest—recommended in treatment of disc problems—will prevent shrinkage and allow full rehydration of the disc. The facet joints in the back must be maintained at a delicate non-weight-bearing relationship for their movement-regulating responsibilities. A well-hydrated disc brings this about by effectively packing the joint, whereas a thin disc will force these joints to become weight-bearing: in the long run, a cause for arthritis—Fig 7.

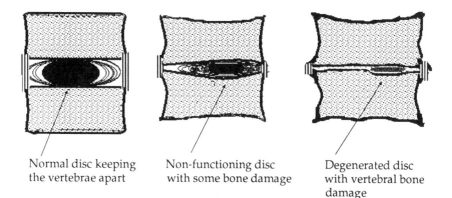

Normal disc keeping the vertebrae apart

Non-functioning disc with some bone damage

Degenerated disc with vertebral bone damage

Fig. 7: *Sketch of the possible progressive stages of disc-associated degeneration of the spinal joints, affecting mainly the lumbar or low back vertebrae.*

Another important effect of disc thickness through adequate hydration is the maintenance of a well-sized aperture or foramen on the side between the two vertebrae, above and below, allowing the nerve to pass through without being squeezed.

The disc is composed of an outer fibrous material and an inner pulpy substance. Between the pulpy substance of the disc and the bone plate of the vertebra lies a layer of cartilage. In fact, a layer of cartilage covers the exposed bone surfaces that come in contact with one another, most particularly at the joint surfaces of the vertebrae, the hands, the arms, and the legs. The property of cartilage is such that it permits for lubrication during the movement of the joints. Cartilage stores a large quantity of water, which gives it the easy gliding and lubricating property it possesses.

It is the property and function of the pulpy substance of the disc to absorb or give up its water. The fibrous part firmly fixes the disc to bony edges of the vertebrae in the back and the sides. These vertical bands of elastic tissue act as "springs" when the disc core that is fully hydrated and expanded presses against them. In front, the fibrous capsule fuses with the bony body of the vertebra, not at its edge, but at the front above the lip, creating a potential anatomical space between the front lip of the vertebra and the fibrous capsule of the disc, which also becomes a part of the long ligament that runs along the whole length of the vertebral column creating the anterior longitudinal ligament—Fig. 4.

Animals run by coiling and springing their spines; their vertebrae are not as weight-bearing as those of humans. In the upright man, this coiling and springing is translated into walking.

In walking, humans leave their body weight on the leg that remains behind when one leg is moved forward. When the forward leg touches the ground, the weight of the body is thrown onto it until the back leg moves. In running, one does exactly the same thing, except that one's weight is thrown forward even before the front leg has touched the ground. This is why the weight of the body increases when running—it has the acceleration of gravity added to it.

The Anatomical Space

The anatomical space allows the vertebrae the freedom of opening and closing in front to make the motion of walking more synchronized; otherwise, if the front lip were fully anchored to the other vertebrae, the motion of the spine would be so jerky and rigid that walking would be very ungraceful. This front lip space also has a further use. Since the disc, other than at the edges, is not fused with the body of the vertebrae, the presence of the space allows a *partial vacuum* to be created. The force of vacuum has several properties. By opening and closing the space, *the vacuum generated will suck water into the disc space*, bringing back what is lost when pressure is brought to bear on the disc nucleus. The force of vacuum also further promotes an *adhesive force* to the components of the joint, making it a supple but firm construction. This is why we speak of the vertebral column as a "coiled spring" —Figs. 1 and 8. A potential cause of disc water loss is standing too long on one's legs or sitting poorly in one position for too long, or slouching in a chair.

It's even worse when you open the back angle of the vertebrae, allowing a directed backward pressure on the disc. This backward pressure could, in the long run, force the disc to move and bring pressure on the nerve or the spinal cord.

The Natural Vacuum in the Disc Space

This force of vacuum can also be the cause of disc problems. If the disc is fully hydrated, the fibrous bands around

19

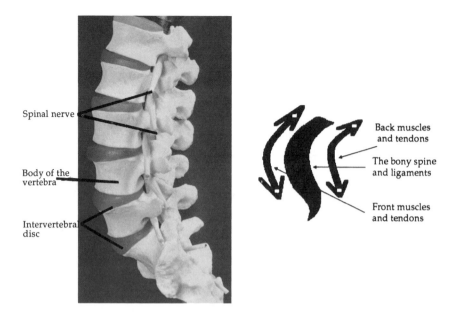

Fig. 8: *The spinal anatomy is made in such a way that the whole structure, although made of many different components, functions as one unit.*

it will maintain a vertical position to take up the pressure of stretching along their whole length; if these bands are not fully and vertically positioned and present a weaker shorter edge, *this adhesive force of vacuum can promote tears in the bands* when undue pressure, such as lifting a weight, causes a greater opening of the back connections of the disc to the vertebrae. Most prone to this phenomenon is the fifth lumbar vertebral disc. The importance of a gentle warm-up before any exercise involving the movement of the spine should become clear.

The importance of water intake on a regular basis for those who have a predisposition to low back pain cannot be stressed enough. Water intake before exercise is also important. You need about one and a half to two liters (approximately one and a half to two quarts) of water a day, even if you don't feel thirsty.

Of course, drinking water will increase your disc efficiency, but how can you take advantage of the knowledge of anatomy and the laws of physics to return your disc to its normal position? It's simple! It's so simple, in fact, that many could not believe the relief of sciatic nerve decompression that resulted in many cases after only half an hour of performing the special exercises using pillows, explained and demonstrated in this manual, even at their first try.

To begin, you must be able to determine that your low back pain has developed into *sciatic pain*.

Chapter 3

Back and Sciatic Pain

If you have had low back pain for some time and now the pain goes down one leg or the other, or even both, you have a fair indication that the pain is from the sciatic nerve, which is under pressure from the disc that has moved as a result of having had the back angle opened up for too long. This pressure can also be from more serious bone problems. If it is from the disc, the two types of exercises demonstrated below can help in a majority of cases that have not become chronic from too long a predisposition to damage or surgery.

A diagnostic method used by professionals is called Lasegue's sign, but a more simple and frequently used method is to see if pressure of the fingertip between the bony posterior processes of the spine or to their sides produces a local pain. This is a good indication that the disc has produced soft tissue pressure on the nerve or the spinal cord which is further aggravated by a pressing of the tissue above the aggravated area. This sign also determines the location and the level of disc protrusion. This sign will also help to monitor the return of the displaced disc to its normal position—Fig 9.

When the posture for reduction is adopted, if the problem is disc displacement, the pain experienced from the pressure of the finger will, in most cases, reduce gradually until it disappears completely. *If the pain has projected into the leg, this pain too will gradually shift upward into the back until it disappears.*

The exercises described below are to be practiced for two purposes. One method using pillows (corrective exercises) has a disc relocation value, *to be used only when there is local pain,* and the others are intended to strengthen the back muscles and promote local circulation to strengthen the fibrous bands and tendons of the area, as well as to rehydrate and realign the discs in their respective spaces. Any one disc problem is an indication that the problem, although to a lesser extent, affects the other discs in the same area. Surgery on one disc is not the answer to this problem, even when the signs point to the involvement of a particular disc. The dehydration damage affects the other discs of the region proportionately. When one disc is removed, the next disc, which now has to bear more of the burden, will become the subsequent problem presenting candidacy for surgery. Cutting through the scar tissues produced after the first surgery predisposes accidental and permanent nerve damage. Some of the people who give in to the attitude of "cut it out and throw it away" will eventually have to go through three or even four surgical procedures; in these, almost always, some damage to the leg nerves results.

For these simple reasons, surgery (in particular) and even injection and repeated manipulation, are *not* satisfactory and natural answers to the problem.

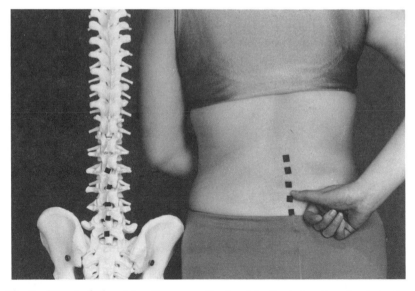

Fig. 9: *How to feel and localize your disc level by the intensity of pain in the region of your spine.*

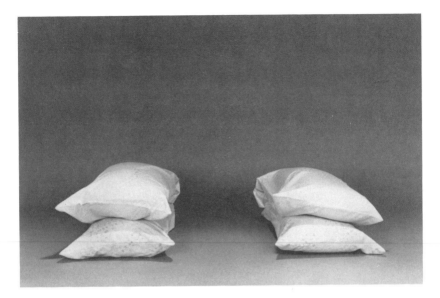

Fig. 10: *The equipment required for the proposed method of bringing the disc back to its normal position: four pillows, placed in the way shown in the picture.*

Corrective Exercises

For the first posture adoption, all you need are four thin pillows. Placed on top of each other (two and two), each set of two should not measure higher than 12 inches—Fig. 10.

Their purpose is to raise your body off the ground about 5 to 6 inches when you lay on them, allowing your back to bend inward slightly and gradually. This is how you open the front angle of your intervertebral spaces, gradually and slowly.

Place the two sets of pillows on the ground, about one and a half feet apart.

Kneel on the edge of the front pillows, with your hands on the ground—Figs. 11A and 11 B.

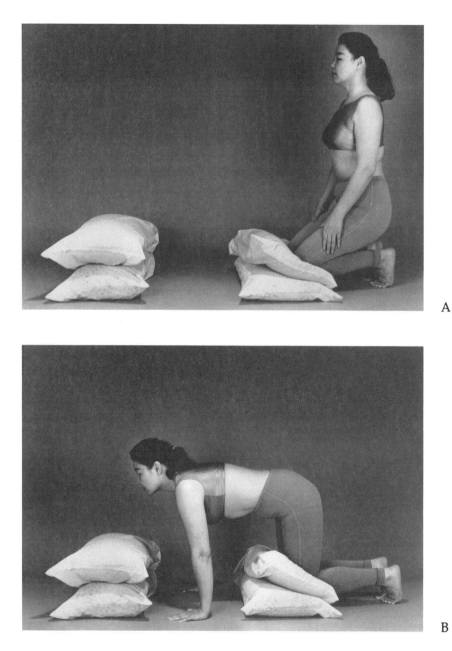

A

B

Fig. 11 A and B: *The initial approach to the corrective position of the body using only four pillows as equipment.*

Now slowly and gently lower your chest until it rests on the front pillows. This will position your abdomen in the hollow between the pillows, allowing your back to bend inwards a little more. Make sure that the area with pain is in the middle between the pillows, allowing a slightly wider opening of the front angle—Figs. 11 C and 11 D.

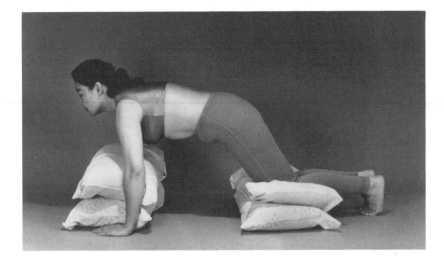

C

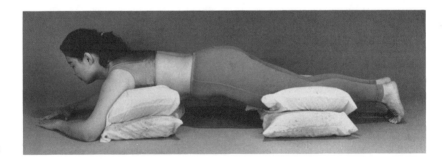

D

Fig. 11 C and D: *The final position on the pillows. Note the potential stiffness that will prevent the back from bending down at first.*

Relax your back by taking deep breaths so that your spine rises up and down; in fact, make sure that the spine is made to move up and down purposely. This is crucial —Figs. 12 A, B, C and 13 A and B.

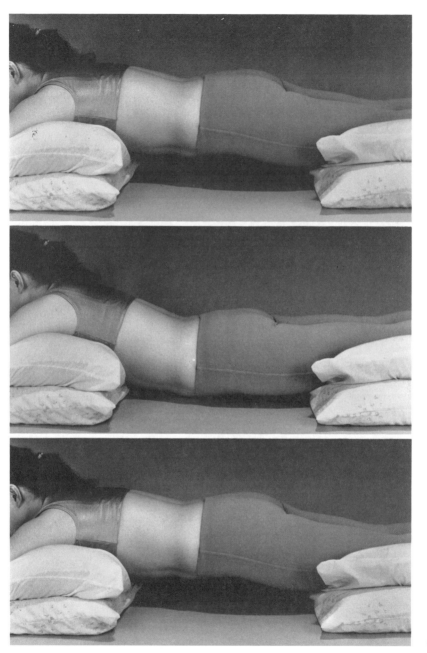

A

B

C

Fig. 12 A, B, C: *Note that all that is involved is a rhythmic movement of the spine in the lower region of the back, producing only one or two degrees of opening and closing of the front part of the intervertebral disc spaces. The human anatomy is designed in such a way that even this small adjustment to posture produces a very significant natural series of events that maintain the normal integrity of the spinal column.*

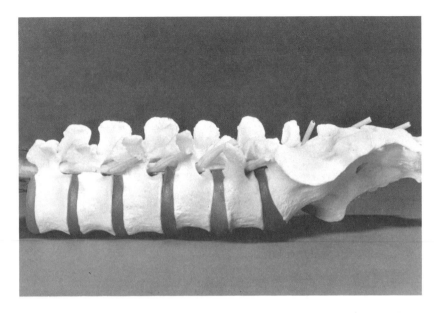

Fig. 13 A: *The anatomical model demonstrating a posture, representing the early rigidity of the spine, shown in figure 11D.*

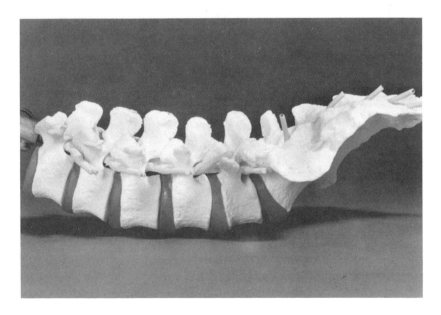

Fig. 13 B: *The anatomical model positioned to show how the very small curvature produced in the spine can effectively open up the front disc spaces.*

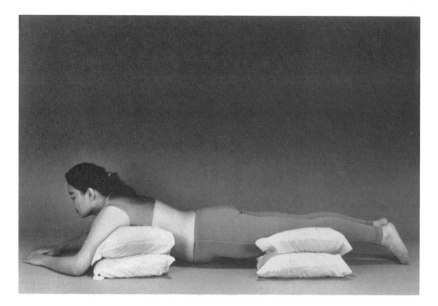

Fig 14: *Note the bend in the back produced after the relaxation that will allow the stomach to reach the ground and open the front disc spaces (see Fig. 13 B).*

While your back may be stiff at the beginning, by this relaxation method your abdomen will now relax and reach the ground—or come very close to it. If, at the beginning, your abdomen is on the ground, you might have to raise the height of the pillows—Fig. 14.

Now that your body is relaxed, after every ten deep inhalations and exhalations, continue normal slow breathing. Now try raising first one leg, then the other, to a comfortable height behind you. Your legs should be raised without bending at the knees. Your toes should be pointing out. The leg should reach as high as possible from behind—Fig. 15. With gradual decompression of the nerve, your leg will have a greater range of movement. The painful spot in your back will become less painful and gradually disappear.

With this movement of the leg, your body will experience a slight rotation at the spinal column—Fig.15. This movement will further encourage the disc to fall back into its hollow position in the body of the vertebra. At times, you can also try to raise both legs when bending your back inward and outward.

You should feel relief as soon as the disc is in its position and local pain is gone. Sometimes it is possible to trace improvement (a lessening) of the sliding pain in the leg if the pain has projected all the way into the leg.

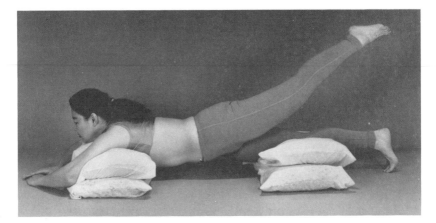

A

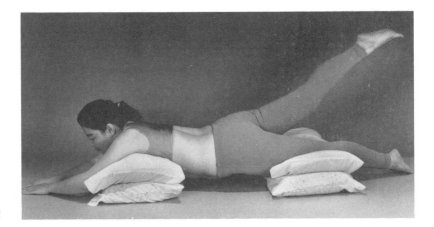

B

Fig. 15: *Pictures showing that alternate raising of the legs produces a natural rotation of the back, intended to relocate the disc to its natural cupped position between the vertebrae—not just the pain-producing disc, but all the lumbar vertebral discs that will have been proportionately affected.*

The taking of deep breaths and raising of the legs should be carried out intermittently until the pain disappears. If you are not successful at first try, a second attempt at a later time might bring forth a better result. *Normally, within half an hour, total relief should result if the condition is disc displacement and you have carried out the instructions correctly.* With a torn disc, the condition might not improve immediately.

The rationale behind this procedure is that the attachment of the front ligament to the disc, by being forced to stretch when the front angle is opened up, will draw the disc back into its intervertebral space and away from the nerve root or the spinal cord. At the same time, by creating a space in the position where the disc used to be, a force of vacuum that will be generated sucks the disc back, along with some water for its rehydration; this force of vacuum will enhance the action of the front ligament in retraction of the disc back to its normal position. The force of vacuum that draws water into the joint will also rehydrate the cartilage covering and separating the bony contact points, enhancing its lubrication and gliding property. Almost all movement-supporting joints benefit from this water-drawing property of vacuum that will be produced during angular movements that stretch the joint. When taking deep breaths, you will also create a stronger vacuum in the abdomen that is also hanging down. The back movement will introduce an intermittent effect, allowing an easier movement of the disc. *The procedure with the pillows need be carried out once or twice and only when there is localized pain.* (For added information refer to the next section of the book.)

Now that you have experienced your first relief from pain, after a few minutes, slide to the side and lay stretched on your abdomen on the ground for a few more minutes, allowing the overstretched ligaments to regain their normal length and strength—Fig. 16.

To get up: Without arching your back, slide backward on your knees. Again without arching your back, bring first one foot under your body, then the other, and rise to your feet. Your walking should now be less painful if you have successfully carried out the procedure and your diagnosis of your own condition has been accurate.

Keep in mind that the information and the procedure you have just learned will help you prevent a deterioration of the pathology associated with back pain. A few glasses of water and a half hour's passive exercise on two pillows will not immediately reverse a chronic problem established over a long period of time. What you have learned so far is good for crisis management; what you now need is persistence with supportive exercises and preventive procedures to avert future crises. You now have the knowledge to handle back pain. *But knowledge by itself is not enough. You will need to act on the information on a daily basis.*

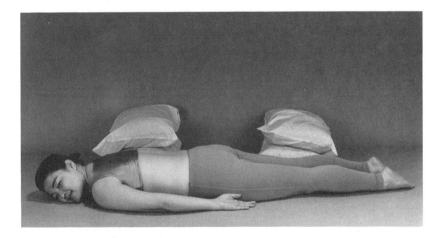

Fig. 16: *Relaxation after the procedure.*

Preventive Exercises

You will now be shown a series of special exercises designed to strengthen your back muscles and, by promoting a better circulation to the area, to bring about the possibility of strengthening the tendons and ligaments, as well as better hydration of the core or the pulp of *all* the vertebral discs and their supportive cartilage separation from the bone.

Muscles that have not been utilized much will, when exercised, develop aches and pains of their own. Although the mechanism is related to the initial back pain, this problem is *not* the same as the initial back pain. This new muscle pain related to the exercise is an indicator that the process of strengthening of the back muscles—and, of course, the tendons and fibrous ligaments—has been established. If the aches and pains are not severe, the exercises should be carried out. If the pain becomes unbearable, an intermission of one or two days might be advisable. However, there is no shortcut or way of strengthening of the soft tissues of the area without exercising. Ultimately, the soft tissues and muscles of the spine *must* be strengthened if relief from back pain is the desired goal.

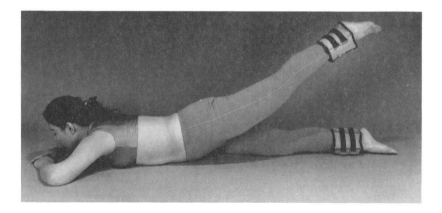

Fig. 17: *Raising one leg and then the other a number of times and eventually using leg weights.*

Lying on your abdomen, raise first one leg and then the other, keeping your toes stretched and the knee straight. Repeat the motion a few times, bringing the raised leg down to rest before you raise the other leg. Remember the number of repetitions you perform so you can increase it gradually with each exercise session. The same applies to all the recommended exercises—Fig. 17.

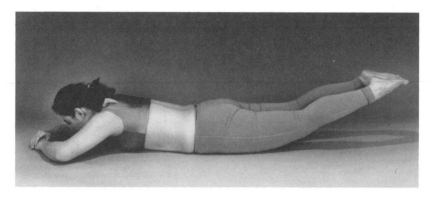

Fig. 18: *Both legs being raised to strengthen all the back muscles.*

Now do the same, bringing both legs up. The movement should be slow and deliberate, knees straight—Fig. 18.

Relax for a few minutes, taking deep breaths to release pressure on your back. With correct exercises, your back will gradually become strong and healthy and you'll never again experience anxiety over the cause of your back pain—Fig. 19.

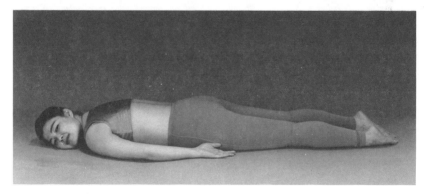

Fig. 19: *Relaxation of the muscles is important.*

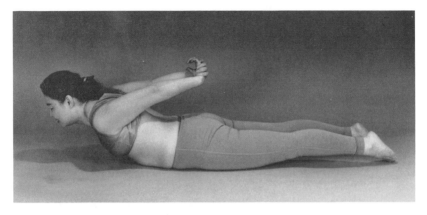

Fig. 20: *The chest vertebrae realignment exercise.*

Now clasp your hands together at the lower back with your elbows bent. Raise your chest as high as you can off the floor and hold it. With your hands still clasped, straighten your elbows and raise your arms away from your body; this exercise forces a contraction of all your back muscles and helps realign the chest and neck vertebrae, a useful exercise for those who suffer from disc problems in the neck region— Fig. 20. Now put the two exercises together; raise the arms and the legs at the same time. Try it five times slowly and purposefully for its exercise value—Fig. 21. Now roll over onto your back and bring your feet in as close to your buttocks as possible—Fig. 22 A.

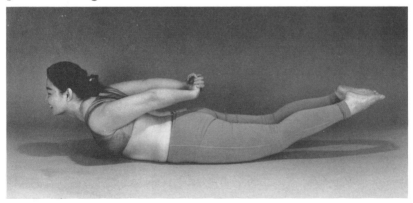

Fig. 21: *The combined exercise to strengthen the back muscles and improve the realignment of the low back, chest, and neck vertebrae with their respective discs.*

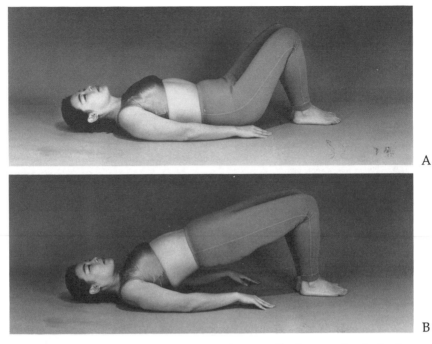

A

B

Fig. 22 A and B: *The initial movements of a very effective exercise for back pain sufferers.*

Keeping this position, raise your buttocks off the ground as high as possible until you feel the pressure in the hollow of your back—Fig. 22 B.

With your pelvis locked up, shift the weight to one foot and raise the other leg off the ground. Remember, keep the knee and the toes straight—Fig. 22 C.

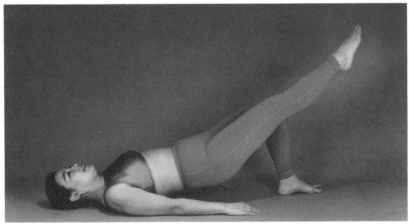

C

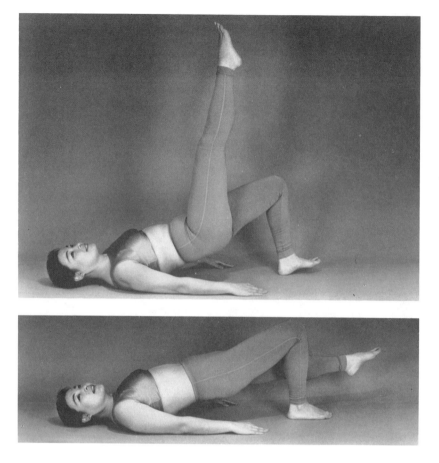

D

E

Fig. 22 C and D: *Back and leg muscles strengthening exercises.*

Continue to raise and lower your leg as low as possible without touching the ground. Do this exercise with each leg about ten times, or less intitially if the pressure on the back muscles is too much—Fig. 22 D and E.

These exercises should be done on a regular basis over a period of time. Eventually you might want to add leg weights to strengthen the muscles, tendons, and the ligaments of the lower back muscles and the abdominal muscles. These muscles are important to a pain-free normal posture of the vertebrae.

A "pot belly" in people who are not fat can be the result of the dehydration of the discs and weak back muscles that cannot keep the vertebral column upright and straight. When the vertebral column develops exaggerated curvatures as a result of weak muscles and less effective discs, the abdomen, which would normally be stretched to stand straight, will not get bone support and will "pot" forward. The above exercises will help those who suffer from this condition.

Now you are better equipped to cope with your low back problems. These exercises will also help your neck discs. In fact, a similar procedure has been helpful in cervical disc problems. All you have to do is rest your forehead or chin on a solid rest (such as a pile of books), neck extended backwards, while going through the deep breathing part of the exercise with your chest on the pillows. Demonstrated exercises (Figs. 20 and 21) are also corrective for neck and chest intervertebral disc displacement.

It should be recognized that the exercises described above have similar corrective influence toward improvement of the condition of back pain sufferers as the sport of swimming. *Swimming is a complementary exercise that should become part of the weekly activity, if it is available.*

Increased water intake and regular exercises to strengthen the back muscles will help the sufferers from the painful condition known as Ankylosing spondylosis (ankylosis).

Precautions

The following precautions are essential:

For the first few days you are trying these exercises, you should not make any back-bending motions or lift heavy objects. If you must lift something, always keep your knees bent and your back upright. Raise the weight by rising on your knees. These cautions are important because your muscle tissue and your ligaments have demonstrated insufficient strength; they need time to regain strength—Fig. 23.

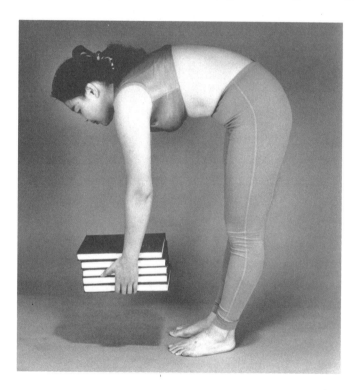

Fig. 23 A: *The wrong way to pick up a load from the ground.*

Avoid soft-spring beds at all costs.

When in motion, try to keep a supple knee movement; *don't* lock your knees during activity that places pressure on your spine.

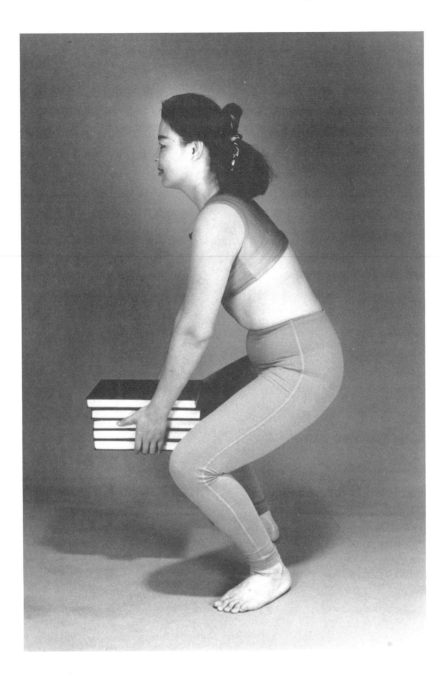

Fig. 23 B: *The correct way to pick up a load from the ground.*

Remember that good posture helps keep the soft tissues strong and the front angle of the vertebrae open, so that the discs will become effective wedges between the vertebrae—Fig. 24.

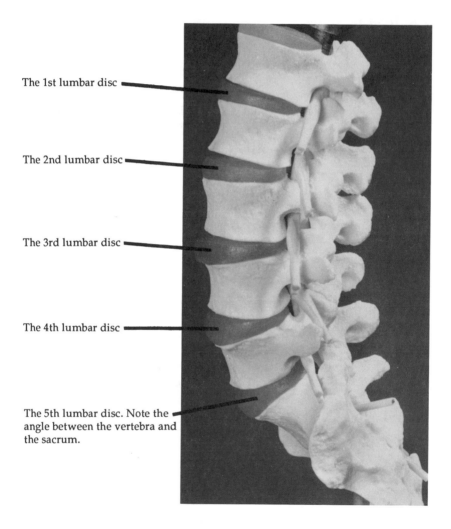

The 1st lumbar disc

The 2nd lumbar disc

The 3rd lumbar disc

The 4th lumbar disc

The 5th lumbar disc. Note the angle between the vertebra and the sacrum.

Fig. 24: *Model of lumbar vertebrae showing the open angle in front, part of the lower curvature of the spine.*

Refrain from too much stooping—Fig. 25.

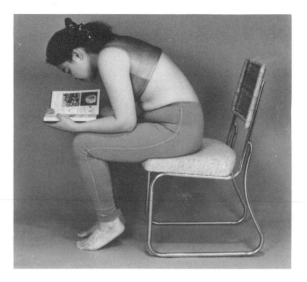

Fig. 25 A: *The wrong posture for working behind a desk or reading a book.*

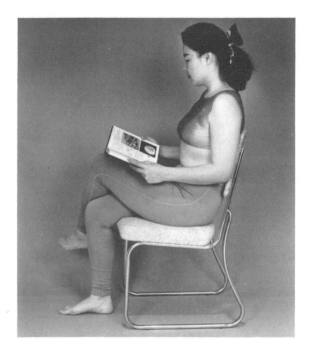

Fig. 25 B: *The correct posture for anyone working for long hours behind a desk.*

Do not sit for too long in an inclined position—Fig. 26.

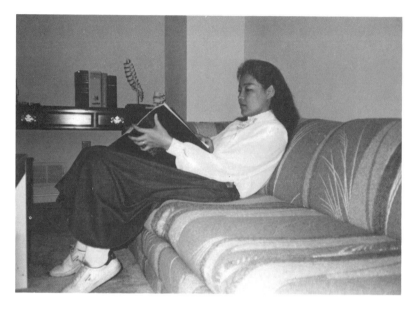

Fig. 26 A: *The wrong position for low back and sciatic pain sufferers.*

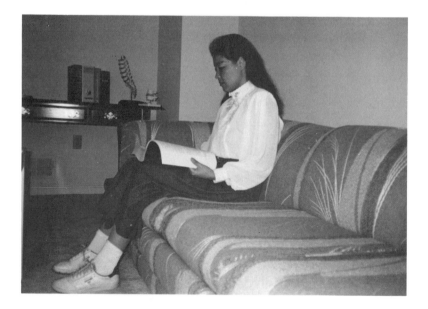

Fig. 26 B: *The correct position for prevention of low back and sciatic pain.*

Congratulations! You have just become one of a small minority who now understands the secrets of the spinal column and its discs and how to make your spine grow stronger and pain-free. *Remember, prevention is nine-tenths of any cure.* If you keep at it, you will not be one of the millions who suffer to the point of needing surgery.

Remember to drink your regular need of water. This will save you from other problems associated with water deprivation of the cells of your body.

Don't underestimate the value of regular exercises, particularly walking, wherein the movement of the large muscle mass helps you keep a stress-free physiology.

Make sure you read the rest of this book. While it contains the same basics for the purpose of revision and for an integrated understanding of the subject, much more detailed information has been incorporated within the different parts of the expanded notes.

The Last Words

Figure 27 (page 46), a sketch highlighting the joint role of water and a series of simple exercises, is designed to permanently paint in your mind the essence of all the information contained in this book.

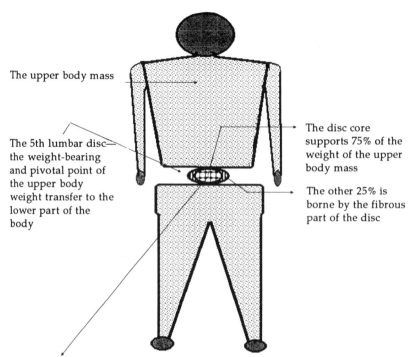

The upper body mass

The 5th lumbar disc—
the weight-bearing
and pivotal point of
the upper body
weight transfer to the
lower part of the
body

The disc core
supports 75% of the
weight of the upper
body mass

The other 25% is
borne by the fibrous
part of the disc

It is the hydrolic property of the disc core that gives it the power to support the weight it has to bear. The disc core consists of living cells that depend on an adequate circulation of serum for their survival and normal function. An adequate daily water intake and proper exercises will establish the normal pattern of circulation through the disc core.

Fig. 27

Welcome Relief

The following letter is included to demonstrate a few points about this simple approach to back problems.

Mr. Winkler's letter is included here to show the length of time I have practiced this method of treating low back problems (my background in the development and refining of the method goes back even further than the letter dates). Mr. Winkler's immediate relief of pain, which had bothered him for some time, was also a joyful experience for him. His understanding of the condition and recognition of the value of selective exercises has maintained his total health, as well as his total relief from back pain all this time.

December 21, 1988
Dr. Fereidun (sic) Batmanghelidj
2146 Kings Garden Way
Falls Church, Virginia 22043

Dear Fereidun (sic):

I am pleased to detail the events leading up to and following your happy suggestion to me in Tehran in 1976 regarding back therapy.

My first experience with back problems came while I was pushing a manual lawn mower up a rather steep hill at my residence in Washington, D.C. in 1971 or 1972. This had followed some months of unsupervised exercise during which I had undoubtedly strained my back. Following the lawn mower incident I saw an orthopedic specialist who, following X-rays, diagnosed a ruptured disk. He set forth a course of exercise which I followed for a while and then gave up. He also said I must sleep on my side in a fetal position or on my back with one or two pillows under my knees.

I arrived in Tehran in the spring of 1973 and shortly thereafter began regular swimming. This helped but I still continued to have sieges of several weeks to several months when I was in considerable pain, was unable to lift anything and gradually got relief through a back brace and restricted activity. During these sieges my body was quite twisted.

It was during one of these attacks that you and I were together at a dinner party and, noticing my twisted condition and obvious discomfort, you suggested a different approach. I told you that I was sleeping only in a fetal position because of the doctors orders. You drew some skeletal diagrams on a piece of paper and advised me to try sleeping on my stomach with a pillow under my chest and another under my thighs. I recall telling you that this totally contradicted the directions I had been given and that I was concerned lest I really damage myself. In any event when Peggy and I went home we discussed your counsel and she said something to the effect of "What can you lose, since you are obviously in terrible pain?" So I tried your method. I could only remain in your rather uncomfortable position for about 45 minutes and was, of course, unable to sleep in the position. You had told me this probaby would be sufficient. It was. The next morning I was fine. Since then I have had fewer and less intense back sieges (although I was once again diagnosed following X-rays by a different Washington orthopedic physician as having a ruptured disk) and each time I try a short period on my stomach with pillows under the chest and thighs. It seems to work. I do credit swimming — four to five miles each week—with a significant contribution to my back situation but whatever the reason, I am able to carry heavy suitcases during the frequent trips we take and am uninhibited by my back.

Sincerely,

Gordon Winkler

47

Dear Dr. Batmanghelidj,   June 24, 1996

On June 29, 1995, I hurt my back. On June 30, 1995, in a lot of pain I called my medical doctor. He was closed and couldn't see me until July 3. On June 30, I went to chiropractor. He took X-rays, gave treatment, and I received some relief.

On July 3, I saw my medical doctor. He examined me, then sent me to a physical therapist for three different days. I had some relief, not much.

Returned to medical doctor on July 10, still in pain. He gave me some more pain pills, he had me take X-ray of lower spine, plus CAT-scan of lower spine. He also sent me back to physical therapist for three more days. Again some relief.

July 13, still in pain. Medical doctor sent me to have MRI on back. Also during this time I had two more chiropractor treatments. During all the above time I was on pain pills twice a day.

My wife remembered reading in Dr. Julian Whitaker's Health and Healing Newsletter (March 1995, Vol. 5, No 3), where he mentioned your book, "How to Deal with Back Pain & Rheumatoid Joint Pain." She went to local bookstore, purchased book for $14.95. We hurriedly read your book, did exercises as you suggested, started drinking water. WITHIN ONE HOUR MY BACK WAS PAIN FREE, and has remained so ever since. God bless you.

What really ticks me off, plus the pain I was in, is:

THE MEDICAL DOCTOR CHARGED FOR HIS 3 VISITS	$150.00
THE PHYSICAL THERAPIST'S SIX VISITS	$651.50
X-RAYS AND CAT SCAN	$209.00
CHIROPRACTOR, X-RAY AND THREE VISITS	$155.00
MRI	$543.50
SANTAIAM MEMORIAL HOSPITAL	$129.00
TOTAL CHARGES WITH VERY LITTLE RELIEF	$1,838.00

Your book and instruction only cost $14.95, and you gave me almost immediate relief in only one treatment.

Again God bless you for your books and knowledge. We now also have your book, "Your Body's Many Cries for Water," your video, your audio tape. They are all exceptional. If you publish anything else I want them.

Sincerely,

Dorman J. Bryce

DORMAN J. BRYCE
4940 Sunnyside Ridge Rd. SE #G6
Salem, OR 97302

Chapter 4

Rheumatoid Joint Pain
(Rheumatoid Arthritis)

When any of your joints—the vertebral joints, the joints of the fingers and the hand, or even the knee and the ankle joints—begin to signal aching pains that come and go, and every time these pains stay longer, the first thought that should occur to you is: "My body is severely short of water." This initial assumption is a "cardinal must." My published clinical and scientific research show that *chronic pains of the body are indicators of chronic dehydration.*

We lose our thirst sensation at a steady rate from the age of 20 onward. As a result, our bodies becomes chronically dehydrated *without being able to recognize the gradually increasing water shortage.* The body has no water storage system to draw on in times of need. If the body needs to shift water for a particular function, initially it draws from the water volume that is inside the cells. Any pure water that you drink will also try to get into the cells. That is to say, it leaves the blood circulation and gradually works its way into the cells.

There is a predetermined pattern for priority distribution of the available water to the essential organs of the body. The liver takes priority; all the food and water intake of the body is initially processed through the liver. The brain, which is more or less 1/50th of the total body weight in an average-sized person, receives between 18 and 20 percent of the total circulation that is fully oxygenated. The lungs receive 100 percent of the unoxygenated blood that also contains 100 percent of the concentration of the food and water supply that has passed through the liver. When the body is short of water, the blood that goes through the lungs is highly concentrated.

Cholesterol

The organs and the anatomical parts that have a ready supply of blood circulation and are on the "direct highway" are less likely to suffer from a water shortage although even these anatomical parts will ultimately receive less and less when the drought in the body continues and becomes a permanently established situation. Cholesterol buildup in the arteries of the body is a component of drought management. Its increased production and presence in the arterial wall is one of the chemical mechanisms for decreased water permeation through the wall of the cells lining the vessels.[6] Increasing the water intake before meals to prevent blood from becoming concentrated will reduce the cholesterol levels in circulation. A substantial water intake (3/4 to one pint) at a time interval of half an hour before meals is astoundingly effective in the reduction of the cholesterol levels in circulation.

Joint Cartilage and Bone Circulation

The anatomical parts that suffer most when there is a shortage of water in the body are those without a direct vascular circulation. The anatomical parts that depend for the supply of their needs on the seepage of tissue fluids through another organ suffer most. They will not receive what they need; the mediating organ will trim its transit routes. The anatomical parts that are excellent examples of this thesis are the joint cartilages (Figs. 28 and 29) and the *intervertebral discs*. I have explained the mechanisms involved in disc hydration. I will now try to explain the basic problem in the feeding of joint cartilage that is the root cause of damage in the rheumatoid joints and their pain signal, be they the finger joints, the knee joints, or the vertebral joints.

Remember, there is no functioning "dead" part in the body

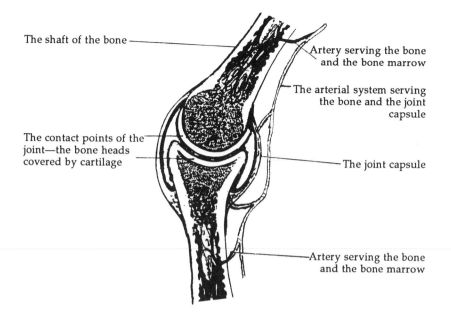

The shaft of the bone

Artery serving the bone and the bone marrow

The arterial system serving the bone and the joint capsule

The contact points of the joint—the bone heads covered by cartilage

The joint capsule

Artery serving the bone and the bone marrow

Fig. 28: *The normal finger joint demonstrating the common arterial supply to the area. The artery to the capsule can dilate to bring increased blood circulation to the soft tissues of the joint. The artery that goes through the bone canal is restricted by the size of its passageway.*

that is nature-designed. All tissues of the body, including bone, cartilage, and even the disc core are composed of *living* cells that have to remain alive and be reproductive of daughter cells (except the brain cells that are not replaced before they die) for that particular organ to function. The dead tissue (cells) is eaten away by the "garbage collectors" and new tissue replaces them. For the tissue to remain alive, the most simple and initial need is water itself, and then whatever food supply the water can bring with it.

The bone connections of the fingers, hands, and most movement-supporting joints are separated by means of cartilage pads that are firmly stuck to the bone. The bone ends to which cartilage is connected are thin, whereas the wall of their shafts are made of solid and thicker tube-like bones. The artery of the bone goes through and divides in the canal systems in the thick section of the bone. The canals in the bone act as though they are straightjackets (Fig. 28) that may not permit dilation of the vessels, even if the vessels themselves could dilate to increase the circulation to the area (the very mechanism that brings greater circulation to the capsule of the joint, whereas the artery that goes through the bone is severely restricted by the fixed size of its canal through the bone). Each bone of the skeleton has only one (very rarely two) artery to feed that bone. Inside the hollow spaces of these bones nature has housed the manufacturing system of the blood cells—red cells as well as all of the variations of white cells. Nature gives priority to the development of these cells, which entirely depend on many different functions of water in particular.[1] When there is dehydration, there will not be enough water to supply the end bone cartilage with its needs—Fig. 29; the blood manufacturing system exercises its priority by means of specially active cation pumps that force the water into the expanding blood cells, which must consist of at least 75 percent water.

Fluid in the Joint

In the soft tissues and cartilage of the joints, very fine—almost single strand—nerves have recently been demonstrated. This indicates that a direct connection between the joint and the nervous system does exist. When the cartilage of the joint cannot get its water and food supply from the bone circulation, the arterial circulation to the joint covering and capsule will begin to dilate (Fig. 29) and have fluid available for its pumping and vacuum suction into the joint when the joint begins to move. There is another masterly design of nature in this process, which is commonly labeled as the *sterile inflammation of the joints* (sterile means non-infectious). Since the circulation to the joint surfaces is sluggish and yet the cartilage cells are living tissue and in need of oxygen, nature has devised an oxygen manufacturing system in some of the inflammatory cells. This local oxygen manufacturing capability has two purposes. Firstly, it acts as an antiseptic against bacteria and, secondly, it provides oxygen for the cells that are floating about or are lodged within the cartilage pads. This is an emergency oxygen supply system to the isolated area of the joint space. The fluid in the joint should not be removed, unless bleeding is suspected. If the fluid is clear, it should be left alone in the joint. Joints that have had their fluid removed (particularly knee joints) do not repair as quickly as joints that are allowed to retain their fluid.

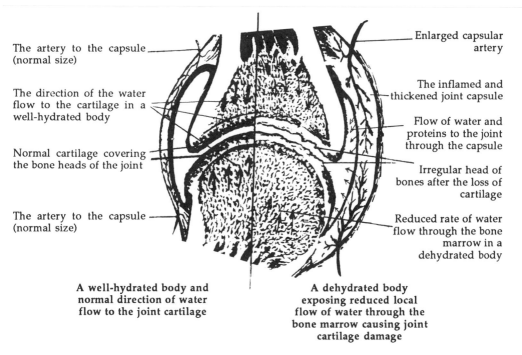

The artery to the capsule (normal size)

The direction of the water flow to the cartilage in a well-hydrated body

Normal cartilage covering the bone heads of the joint

The artery to the capsule (normal size)

Enlarged capsular artery

The inflamed and thickened joint capsule

Flow of water and proteins to the joint through the capsule

Irregular head of bones after the loss of cartilage

Reduced rate of water flow through the bone marrow in a dehydrated body

A well-hydrated body and normal direction of water flow to the joint cartilage

A dehydrated body exposing reduced local flow of water through the bone marrow causing joint cartilage damage

Fig. 29: *The left side of the figure represents a normal flow of "water" and nutrient needs of the cartilage covering of the joint bones. The right side represents a decreased flow of "water" to the cartilage covering through the bone. The arterial supply to the capsule becomes increased, causing swelling and effusion into the joint. This route of supply of nutrients is not completely effective for the growing end of the cartilage covering the bones. Forced activity of the joint will damage the cartilage and leave the bone exposed and permanently damaged.*

Equally important is the intelligent restriction in the use of anti-inflammatory medications, particularly those that tamper with the local oxygen manufacturing capability of the inflammatory cells.

Most initial joint pains disappear after some movement; the natural vacuum created by the movement of the joint may be the mechanism for joint hydration from the vessels in the soft tissue joint covering. However, for the act of dilation and shunting of circulation, the agents involved also produce pain. The pain signal indicates three points: one, that the area or the joint is dehydrated and does not get its fluid requirements from its bone route of supply; two, that the shunting system to bring water and food to the joint is in operation; three, that the joint should not be used until full hydration of the joint has taken place and the joint cartilage, which has a high wear-and-tear rate, can be repaired from its base. This latter cardinal point should be taken seriously.

The Cartilage Repair System

The repair system of the cartilage can only be established from the base cells that are attached to the bone. The contact surfaces that rub against one another, even when water and food supply are now made available to them, cannot provide the permanent padding that normally develops from the bone-connected growing base of the cartilage. If the signals of water deficiency of the joint cartilage are not recognized for what they mean, and pain-killers of whatever kind are used, no matter how pretentious to providing the solution, the immediate outcome will be a dependence on the addictive medication. The more important result of this inaccurate and bad education will be that *permanent* damage to the cartilage separation of the joint bones will develop. The cartilage will die in places and the bone surface will be exposed to direct contact.

This is when osteoarthritis and joint deformity will be established—an irreparable joint pathology (Fig. 29). A far more important problem can be the dangerous side effects of these chemical medications. They can produce chemical-physiological complications that in extreme cases may eventually cause death, often from severe bleeding into the stomach. Every year, thousands die from this very complication of the use of "pain-killers" in rheumatoid arthritis.

Rheumatoid Joint Pain: A Signal of Dehydration

The human body is the result of a "well knit together" myriad of systems. We should think of the body as a tight package of many, many different systems that are *bound together by the hidden powers of water;* much like society is bound together by its monetary system. In the same way that the indicators of depression in the oil industry or the housing industry are a sign that the total economy of the country will be affected, the water shortage that has produced signals at the finger joints is also an indicator that other systems of the body will sooner or later signal their damaged state.

There is a gap between the ongoing effect of dehydration and the signal-producing stage of the same dehydration, very much like a company that runs short of cash flow and needs to trim its activity and lay people off when it can no longer continue and has to borrow money or declare bankruptcy. The finger joint is like a company that is a member of a conglomerate. When it runs short of water, it has to borrow from the other members of the conglomerate. However, the conglomerate has an efficient distribution system that has been aware of this local need and has provided the joint with what water it can spare. These compensatory steps are carried out at an automatic and imperceptible level that the conscious mind is not aware of. However, it is almost always the conscious mind that places on the joints of the hand or the legs the burden of movement beyond their rationing supply and capacity to endure. The pain signal is an alert system for the conscious mind to curtail its demands until it attends to the *correct translation* of the chronic pain signal of the joint unit of the conglomerate "body."

Medical science, having taken its lead from the science of chemistry, has concentrated totally on the 25 percent solid matter of the body and has stubbornly—and possibly self-ishly—ignored the all important role of the 75 percent water content. The medical practitioners are not fully aware of the signal systems associated with body water mal-regulation and metabolism. However, the broader aspects of this discrepancy have been exposed; if they choose to investigate the scientific statements on this topic, the practice of medi-cine will transform in favor of the patient in a very short period of time. Until such time that the above-mentioned scientific logic penetrates the everyday practice of medicine by the professionals, individual patients will need to educate *themselves* on their body's signals of dehydration.

Rheumatoid joint pain is a direct signal of local water deficiency of the body. If water intake is consciously and regularly adjusted to the needs of that particular body, in most cases, these pains will gradually disappear. The local swelling of the joint surfaces will possibly disappear too. What is more important, the joint structure will begin to repair itself, if gross deformity has not already been estab-lished.

Even more important than these advantages, the total physiology and all the other organs of the body will benefit from a correct translation of this body water deficiency signal. Different bodies have different types of first "call" for water shortage. If you have not had any other type of "call" signal or indication of water shortage of your body, and you now have chronic rheumatoid joint pain, you should assume that your body's priority shunting system for circulation give its indicators for water shortage from the joints that are now placing a greater demand on the body water supply. In your case, joint pain (rheumatoid) that has no other good reason to be there (injury, infection) should be assumed to be one of the initial thirst signals of your body.

If the professionals who treated the poor child psychiatrist mentioned in Chapter 1 had the above information in addition to their generated arsenal of false knowledge on the curative effect of anti-inflammatory drugs used in rheumatoid arthritis, she might have been saved from the devastating impact of dehydration in her body at a much earlier and manageable stage of her health problems. These problems, as you recall, eventually complicated the lives of the other members of her family to the point of their total extinction.

The Simplest of All Solutions

You should drink no less than one and one half to two liters of water (roughly one and one half to two quarts) every day. This volume of water should be taken throughout the day: one full glass half an hour before each meal and one full glass two and one half hours after each meal, the remainder to be divided between the early morning and the afternoon or the evening.

This approach to water intake also has *proven* clinical merit in the treatment of peptic ulcer disease. I have successfully treated more than 3,000 peptic ulcer sufferers with the above water regimen (the dyspeptic pain signal is another thirst signal of the human body). The references to these statements are included in the list of references at the end of the book.

It should also be recognized that even with adequate water intake, the process of full rehydration of the body is slow. It can take some time before the total cellular rehydration can establish. In any event, thirst sensation must always be satisfied by an increase in water intake, even if the recommended regimen for water intake is observed regularly. With increased water intake, the thirst sensation becomes more sensitive to the dehydration of the body.

March 18, 1996

Dr. F. Batmanghelidj, M.D.
% Global Health Solutions
PO BOX 3189
Falls Church, VA 22043

Dear Dr Batmanghelidj;

I'm responding to your request for information on how your book <u>Your Body's Many Cries for Water</u> helped me.

Enclosed find a book report I wrote for my newsletter, <u>Straws in the Wind</u>. The report is self-explanatory, but I want to update you in as much that I continue to be pain-free with my ankylosis spondylitis one year after starting the water/salt regime. My blood pressure is normal, as well.

I thank God every day for allowing me to finally be pain-free, thanks to Dr Batmanghelidj great book. The Mayo Clinic told me back in 1965 that there "was no cure for my form of arthritis." I would appreciate it if you would forward a copy of this letter (and book report) to them, in the hope that they will finally wake up to the fact that there is a cure for ankylosis spondylitis.

The paradigm shift is on, and if the Mayo Clinic doesn't want to get caught up in the dust cloud, they'd better get with the program.

Who ever said we don't have any modern day heroes? Dr Batmanghelidj is mine!

May God bless you doctor.

Sincerely,

Lloyd Palmer
Lloyd Palmer
Editor/Publisher
<u>Straws in the Wind</u>

> *This letter is reproduced here to show that, even after 30 years, the excruciating pain of ankylosing spondylitis (arthritis of the spinal column) can be cured with water and some salt.*

Chapter 5

Expanded Notes on
Posturally Created Natural Force
of Intermittent Vacuum within the
Intervertebral Disc Spaces

*A Scientific Explanation for a Series of
Special Exercises* ©

To enhance the educational approach of this manual, and with the intention of expanding on the brief information given in the preceding pages, to maintain continuity of thought, the basic principles behind this approach to treatment of low back pain are explained once again, and more information is included.

Posturally Created Natural Force of Intermittent Vacuum within the Intervertebral Disc Spaces

A Scientific Explanation
for a Series of Special Exercises

This self-treatment manual, by dealing with the knowledge of physiology, logic of anatomy, and the laws of physics, can become a guide to your relief, a safeguard from confusion, and protection from misrepresentation. Without detracting from its true value, this manual can afford to be brief because it deals with the application of these sciences to a simple and preventable problem.

The method of postural intervertebral disc realignment and the scientific explanations presented below are the result of many years of research. This method of postural reduction of the prolapsed disc is the result of over 25 years of privately practicing the procedure. Initially, the writer had to deal with his own sciatic pain and eventual paralysis of his right leg. The scientific explanations are the result of more than 10 years of full-time research into the phenomenon of pain, two years and seven months of it spent on clinical evaluation of the effect of water on the condition normally classified as peptic ulcer disease. This was followed by well over eight years of constant theoretical research into the physiology of pain—not the techniques of pain evaluation, but the reasons for its occurrence.

The writer has been publishing his scientific views in the professional journals (see bibliography). It is essential now to provide the same simple explanations on the meaning of chronic pain to the public. It is the sick and the suffering public who desperately need a simplified version of the information provided to the professionals so that they can liberate themselves and their physicians from the conflict of interest that has converted the noble art of healing into "The Health-Care Industrial System," a totally commercial approach to medicine that will destroy the fabric of society (in more ways than one) if allowed to go its merry way. The scientific solution and explanations offered are simple. It is the public and those who suffer from chronic pain who are the ultimate judges of the usefulness of the knowledge presented in this volume of the series on health education.

This book is the first in a series that will attempt to give simple explanations on medical conditions to the layman who would like to understand his or her own problems and take precautions, and to know when to consult a professionally qualified person to investigate his or her problem.

The purpose of this book should not be confused. What is being presented is information about a common problem that may benefit many sufferers. If you are sure your problem of backache and sciatic pain involves your disc degeneration, the following information will help you. If there are other physiological disturbances that appear to mimic a disc problem, and obvious improvement does not follow upon carrying out these simple precautionary procedures, then it is advisable to seek professional help.

What Is Pain?

Neurophysiologists classify "pain" as a sensation. Clinicians try to evaluate the meaning of this "sensation" according to its location, intensity, and duration. Recently, it has been suggested that the subjective explanations of the patients are not enough for a basic evaluation of pain. It is being said that the interpretation of the sufferer is not good criteria for pain evaluation. Now charts and scales are being drawn up and each complaint may have to be read against a "scale." Once again, an individual's sensation of pain will have to fit statistical criteria to develop importance. In other words, the perceptive powers are abandoned and a more "visual" approach is sought, and if your condition does not fall within a statistical norm, then you either "imagine" you are feeling pain or your condition is an aberration from the norm and therefore not suitable for the adopted current methods of evaluation and treatment.

We will not become involved in any of these arguments. Rather, following are my views on what "pain" is and, briefly, how it is caused. For more detailed information, the reader can refer to the references listed.

Sources of Back Pain

1. From the soft tissue

a. Directly related to the vertebral column, such as muscles, tendons and ligaments;

b. Tissues and organs not related to the vertebral column, such as the kidney, appendix, and other structures.

2. From bone involvement

a. Primary inherited abnormalities of the bone structure of the vertebral column;

b. Chronic or overuse problems, such as facet joint degeneration;

c. Acute injury such as fractures, etc.

Over 80 percent of all back pains begin with muscle spasm. The other 20 percent or less have possibly reached a more serious stage of the basic problem.

In this book, the problem of low back pain, an indicator of soft tissue dysfunction leading to eventual problems of disc degeneration and subsequent damage to the bone structure of the region, will be briefly explained.

The Cell

All organs and tissues of the body consist of individual cells. These cells are subgrouped together to form the variety of structures of the body. Any cell, no matter where, while retaining its basic properties, develops only a subspeciality of function in keeping with the particular character and requirement of the tissue in question.

All cells of the body have an outer membrane or "skin." This membrane isolates the contents of the cell and prevents it from mixing with the fluid or solution environment of the cell. In the circulatory system, this fluid is blood (one type of tissue in itself); outside the blood vessels, it is the interstitial fluid that surrounds the cell.

The primary function of the fluid around the cell is to act as a solvent to the minerals, which exist in their ionic form (the purest form of the element): food in the form of amino acids, sugar and carbohydrates and obviously oxygen carried to the cell. It is also a solvent and a transport system for the byproducts of cell metabolism and manufactured substances. The minerals—such as sodium, potassium, calcium and magnesium, often called cations (cat-i-ons)—are maintained in a finely regulated equilibrium between the intracellular (inside the cell) compartment and the extracellular (outside the cell) space.

Much of the energy and function of cells is determined by the rate of movement of these minerals in and out of the cells in a liquid environment. We have inherited these properties of cell function from the earlier cells living in the "primeval soup" during the phase of life in water. It is almost the identical fluid environment and a similar telescoped period that a fetus goes through during its intrauterine phase of creation, except that the fetus gets food and oxygen through its umbilical cord.

Acidity and the Cell

We have all, at one time or another, suffered from muscle fatigue and the pain that follows. We are told pain is caused by excessive lactic acid (under the same circumstances, phosphoric acid, potassium and *histamine* are also excessively found) within the muscle tissue. The lactic acidosis is brought about when muscles are used beyond their oxygen supply or sufficient blood circulation in the region to institute the compensatory processes needed to reestablish physiological homeostasis. *Homeostasis* means functional equilibrium within a norm.

Acidosis and alkalosis are the two ends of a very delicate balancing act in the body to prevent tipping the balance towards the higher reading of the two ends of the scale. The scale is read against acid or hydrogen ions and/or alkali or hydroxyl ions. Seven to one is acid (one is the more acid end of the scale). Seven is neutral, and seven to fourteen is alkali (fourteen is the more alkali end of the scale). This scale is called the pH scale. The pH, or the concentration of the hydrogen ion in the body is, by and large, on the alkali side. The inside content of the ordinary cell (cytosol) is always on the alkali side of the scale, around 7.4. When this number changes toward the acid side, and many cells suffer from this change, a comparative *acidosis* will have taken place. We normally talk of acidosis when the pH of blood changes towards more acidity. But it is also possible to have a *regional acidosis* when there is low circulation to an active region, such as the muscle tissue or the fibrous tissue excessively used.

The Nerves Sensitive To Pain

All the tissues of the body are supplied with nerve endings or so-called *nerve supplies*. These nerve endings could be for motor regulation and maintenance of posture, or for evaluation of the senses: heat, touch, and pain. Presumably we have all heard of *adrenaline*, and the *adrenergic* system, and of *acetylcholine* and the *cholinergic* system within the central and the peripheral nervous tissue. We also have to be aware of another system, called the *serotonergic* system, with *serotonin* as its transmitter agent. It is now agreed more and more that all pain sensations are evaluated within this system in the brain. Even narcotics such as morphine and heroin register their effects through manipulation of this system.

The serotonergic system is well represented in all tissues of the body: in the skin, joints, muscle, vascular bed and, in fact, extensively in the brain structure itself. Its role in the regulation of the physiology of the body and the coordination of all the different functions within other systems is now being recognized and evaluated. It is proposed that the serotonergic nerve endings become sensitized to the pH change in the region of high activity when the circulation is inadequate to sufficiently hydrate the cells, i.e., maintain the various functions of the cell toward homeostasis. This same system is also responsible for registration of heat changes.

Agents Causing Pain

There is a substance (enzyme) in the body called *pre-kallikrein* (pre-kali-krine). A local change in pH can convert this substance to *kallikrein;* kallikrein then converts *kininogens* to *kinins*. Kinins, when brought across nerve endings, can cause pain.[18] It is proposed that this phenomenon is responsible for pain associated with lactic acidosis of muscle tissue, should this be in the untrained muscles of the leg after prolonged exercise or the lumbar vertebral muscles when maintaining an unchanging posture, or a posture employing a particular set of muscles beyond their capacity for endurance (for example, continuous attempt by the back muscles at correcting the bad posture of the upper part of the body against the force of gravity). The natural purpose behind creation of kinins is to dilate the local vessels and to increase the local circulation; at the same time, they decrease the local activity by producing pain.

An inherent characteristic of any living tissue is a constant drive to maintain a finely regulated buffered pH (neutral around 7.4). Since the cell membrane of any tissue is an ionic barrier, to keep a regulated pH, ionic pumps have been devised by nature. Each cell, depending on its functional requirement, may have up to several thousand of these pumps. These pumps are complex proteins, each with a special affinity for any particular pairs of ions. Recently published research reports have demonstrated that a particular pump exchanges hydrogen ions for sodium ions.

One of the important characteristics of these pumps is the property of the ions' buildup on the "intake side" that becomes the starter or the switch to the pump drive. This means that if there is an increase in the hydrogen ion (acid) in the cell, the pumps begin to increase function, i.e., hydrogen ion(acidity) will leave the cell and sodium ion will enter the cell. These pumps need to do a balanced work; when something is carried out, another substance has to replace that element and therefore must be carried into the cell.

There are other pumps doing exactly the same type of work, except that now sodium ions are exchanged for potassium ions; sodium is taken out of the cell and potassium is pushed back into the cell. The calcium ion in the body is also similarly regulated. These pumps regulate the electrolyte and ionic balance of the tissues of the body, essential for all functions within the cells, including maintenance of the normal density of bone structure.[6]

Free Water

No active function takes place within the body without expenditure of energy (conversion of ATP). It seems that the energy transformation for this pumping action is brought about by "free water."[11]

Water in the body is found in two different forms. There is *osmotically bound* or "inactive water" (water that is busy with some other material) and there is *osmotically active* or "free water"[12] (water that can be engaged to do new work). It is this free water that becomes the energy-inducer for these cation or ionic pumps.[11]

In the body, this free water has the same value that a healthy cash flow would have in a business establishment— that is, it "gets things done." With increased availability of free water, these pumps become more effective in establishing ionic equilibrium.

It is becoming more and more obvious that the thirst sensation is not a reliable fine regulator of body water content, and with increasing age this sensation becomes even more unreliable.[6, 23-25] A state of chronic dehydration can exist without the body recognizing it, to the extent that the cells of the body will become comparatively dryer than before. Under such conditions, the "free water" content of the body may not be sufficient to operate these cation pumps effectively to maintain optimum function. In such circumstances the buildup of hydrogen ion in the tissue, having used more of its free water than its ability to replace, will cause pain. Such pain should indicate a "free water" deficiency, and therefore a form of *tissue thirst*.

This type of pain should be treated with increased regular intake of water—no less than about a liter and a half of water a day, even when one is not thirsty. Attention to this recommendation is absolutely essential, since with increase in age we tend to lose function within these "dryer" cells. It is this gradual change in the ratio of "free water" inside the cells compared to water outside the cells that brings about aging and loss of function until we die. At age 20, the ratio of water outside the cells compared to water inside the cells is around 0.8 to 0.9, as opposed to age 70 when the ratio becomes about 1.1. I can assure you this vast change is incompatible with efficient cell function in the "dryer regions." All of this comes about as a result of not feeling thirsty enough to optimally hydrate all the cells of the body throughout life. The discs suffer most in this situation, because the discs do not have a blood circulation system to supply them with nutrients and oxygen. Since the cells in the disc structure are also living cells, they need nutrients to continue to function.

With the clear serum fluid being pumped *out* by the pressure of the weight of the body and drawn *in* by osmotic force and vacuum force, a type of circulation takes place in the disc tissue. By taking regular drinks of water, diluting the blood, you will add to the absorbing osmotic force of the disc substance, and therefore a greater chance of full hydration of the disc core.

With increased hydration, the body's proteins and enzymes function much more efficiently,[38] and therefore tissue maintenance and repair will be carried out more effectively.

In Conclusion: Low back pain should be treated with an increase in daily water intake. This type of pain, originating in the soft tissues of the region, has to be taken as an indicator of inadequate fluid and nourishment needed for normal function of this part of the anatomy.[6] Exercise will increase the circulation of water and nutrients to the region.

Referred Pain and/or Muscle Weakness Caused by a Prolapsed Intervertebral Disc

The human body is a unique physical structure. When one considers the laws of gravity, the weight of a body, and the weight-bearing points of the body in constantly altering angles of posture during motion, one must admit to the ownership of a complicated machine! It is a machine that employs an inherent understanding of the laws of physics and chemistry and gives an unhindered passage to one's resolve and drive. It enables one to convert solid matter one eats to ideas and ideals—an altogether astounding phenomenon, when you think of it. But one must also take care of that machine; after all, it is made up of delicate, soft, and fragile components.

One such class of delicate, soft, and fragile components in the body is the weight-bearing, shock-absorbing, joint-packing parts known as *discs*. There are now some 24 single vertebrae and 23 soft discs between these 24 bony structures.

At any given time, more healthy people are prone to disc trouble than any other health problem. Disc lesion is a worldwide problem. Disc problems either send a patient to a medical professional or to an osteopath, chiropractor, or physical therapist. The solutions offered are either surgery for severe conditions or manipulation; in some cases bed rest may be the patient's accepted choice, depending on the severity of the condition.

70

In either of these cases the course of treatment does not show a precise understanding of the physiology of the disc to offer a logical solution in keeping with the complicated ways the disc's existence became essential to the vertebrate animal. This is especially true for the vertebrates that changed posture from the quadruped to the erect two-legged humans. In the erect and upright anatomy of the human body, the disc is a truly weight-bearing component of the vertebral column, whereas in the quadruped the discs do not have to bear the greater part of the weight of the animal.

Fortunately, the distinctive anatomical formation of the spine inherited by man has the same safety mechanisms incorporated in its structure as the quadrupeds possess. Possession of knowledge of this anatomical distinction should help man to maintain and utilize his intervertebral discs to their full capacity without undue suffering and fear. Let us see how!

The Vertebral Column

Before we get involved in the detail, let us touch base with some of the components involved in the anatomy of the vertebral column and their mode of function.

There are seven vertebrae in the region called the neck, 12 in the region called the thorax or chest, and five in the region called the lumbar or lower part of the vertebral column. Anatomically, the sacrum, which joins the two sections of the pelvis, used to be vertebrae but they have now fused together to form one solid and very important connection between the lowest lumbar vertebra and the pelvic girdle. The anatomical vestige of a "tail" is represented by a number of tiny bead-like bones attached to the lower end of the sacrum; these are called *coccyx* (kok-six). These tiny "beads" provide support to the soft tissue around the rectum. If you look at Fig. 1

(page 11), you will see the proportion of the different regions of the vertebral column.

Two other points should also draw your attention. One is the different regional curvatures of the spine and the other is the proportionate change in size of each vertebra from the neck downward. I will later explain the significance of the curvatures, but the reason for the variation in size of the vertebrae is the necessary adaptive change to the weight-bearing requirement. The first cervical (neck) vertebra has to support the "physical" weight of the head, whereas the lowest lumbar vertebra has to support the weight of the head, neck, chest, and the contents of the abdomen—a major proportion of the body's weight. Accordingly, as we look down the column, the lower vertebrae have to become wider and thicker to endure the weight of the increasing mass piled on each disc and the vertebral bone surface.

The Wisdom of Nature

However, that is not the entire story. These bones need to cater to forces much greater than the actual mass weight of the structure they support. With motion, this weight force increases, depending on the type of motion. In running, this force is increased to almost two and one-half to three times its original value. According to the laws of physics, there is an equal and opposite reaction to every action. Therefore, every time a vector or arrow of force is passed down the column, as soon as it reaches the foot and passes on to the ground under the foot (as a mirror reflects light), an equal vector of force will begin to pass up the various solid structures toward the head, except that now this vector represents the sum total of the weight of the whole body, *plus* its multiplier of movement. The usual jargon for this phenomenon is "reactive force."

Fortunately, nature is wise—it is a perfect engineer. Otherwise, if the force of seventy kilos (165 pounds) were to pass down and gather momentum and move up, the brain tissue in the skull would become pulverized after a few steps. Nature has solved the problem by creating counterbalancing curvatures at every level of the body to dissipate the forces that pass through the bone structures. This is the marvel of engineering employed in the design of such a complicated machine—and all of that from single cells, and with such an astounding ability to cope with wear and tear and self-maintenance for so many years of use!

Let us now see how nature solves the problems created by the weight of the body during motion.

Weight and Motion

We have all played with a ball of some kind during our lifetimes. Suppose we release a ball from our hand, allowing it to fall freely to the ground. It will hit the ground and bounce upward, reaching a height less than its original free-fall position. After several up and down bounces, the ball will come to rest on the ground. Depending upon the hardness of the ground and the tension in the ball, some of the energy generated by the impact is absorbed by the ground and the structure of the ball. That is why the ball does not rise to the full height. A heavy stone, on the other hand, when released, would absorb and share the force with the ground. A fragile object such as glass would break.

The human body is not exempt from the same natural laws applying to the ball, the stone, or the glass. An exception that the human body has developed is the ability to dampen the energy of impact in its foot and its arches, in its hip (through the cantilever properties installed in the structure as a result of the position of the hip joint and the spinal attachment to the pelvis), through the circular structure of the pelvic bones (through the elastic and cushion effect of the discs between the vertebral bones), and, finally, through the "coiled spring" properties of the curvatures in the spinal column (Fig. 1, page 11). Let us see how this is done.

The Foot and Its Arches

One of the most important functional roles of the foot, aside from being the point of contact between the ground and the body mass, is its bar spring properties. Figure 5 (page 14) shows the points of contact between the front and back of the foot and the ground. Connecting these two points—and holding the foot in an arched position—is a thick band or fibrous ligament acting as a tension-absorbing spring, enforcing a damping effect on the force of body weight to the ground, and from the ground upward. Thus, the force of weight in motion becomes much less transmittable. This is the reason why people with flat feet find walking and running very difficult. This is also why constant attention to the arch of the foot, through footwear selection, is essential.

Pelvic Anatomy and Distribution of Forces

If you have ever had an interest in target shooting, you would readily appreciate that the material behind the target receiving the bullets must have special characteristics, for if the impact of the bullet is allowed, time after time, to penetrate one spot, before long the material will sustain destructive damage. Knowledgeable inventive minds have thought about the problem and devised a specially designed receptacle with an integrated series of spiral shapes which deflect the bullet, giving it a circular motion until it comes to rest. The force of the bullet does not establish sufficient surface impact to cause damage.

This is a natural physical phenomenon: If a vector of force reaches an object with a circular shape, the force will be continuously deflected. The human body uses this law of nature to its finest detail at every point where force has to be deflected. The best and most successful example of this engineering art is found in the construction of the skull.

It is used also in the construction of the pelvis and in the construction of the discs, where direct force must be dealt with all the time. If you look at Fig. 6 (page 15), you will see the shape of the pelvic girdle and the rough indicators of the way force becomes distributed and breaks up into smaller vectors; at the same time as the force of weight generates energy downward, the impact of that force from the ground generates a vector of force going upward through the vertebral column. These forces are minimal at rest and greatly increased during jumping, running, and walking.

The greatest impact of this weight force distribution is brought to bear on the lumbar vertebral region, the area that has to cope most and the area that suffers most—Fig. 27(page 46). This is why the reader needs to understand the broad highlights of his/her anatomy, to appreciate the reasons for such fine detail in this area, and to realize how easily it is possible to maintain normal function. The body, by adopting these definitions, has been successful in achieving its own transformation from walking on all fours to the more practical upright posture.

The Relationship of the Disc to the Vertebra

A look at Figs. 2, 3, and 4 (pages 12 and 13) will show a number of points.

The vertebra has a body and a projection or lever, called a spine, extending to the back. These spines from each vertebra are joined together by thick fibrous bands, called ligaments and muscle, and they also have bony bearing points on either side. These spines, before they join the body of the vertebra, divide into a v-shaped fork, which joins the body of the vertebra at the two sides. The result is a canal formed at the back of the body. Fibrous bands and sheaths, by joining the bony parts of one vertebra with the others above and below, create a fully covered and strongly protected canal which houses the spinal cord and the nerve roots on their way to the tissues under their control, bathed in cerebrospinal fluid filling the canal space.

Figs. 2 and 3 (page 12) roughly illustrate the relationship of the vertebra's anatomy to that of the spinal cord. The body of the vertebra has a slightly hollow shape which cups the disc from below and roofs the disc from above.

Fig. 3 (page 12) shows the hole through which the individual nerves that separate from the spinal cord pass through the fibrous seal forming the side of the long canal, and extend from the neck to the last vertebra of the back. This canal protects the most vital anatomical part of the body and the cerebrospinal fluid that bathes the nervous tissues (brain and the spinal cord). The nerve passing through the foramen (or the hole on the side) and the spinal cord in the canal seem to become vulnerable to disc problems. If these structures, which are very delicately positioned, alter position and impinge on the soft and sensitive nerve tissue, depending on the extent of the imposition, they can cause localized or referred pain, with progressive deterioration, even paralysis, of the muscles being served by the nerves.

What Is the Disc and What Does it Do?

Figs. 3 and 4 (pages 12 and 13) will give you an idea of the position and the relationship of the disc with the vertebrae. The disc is made up of a very strong fibrous outer cover called the *anulus fibrosus* and an inner softer pulp called *nucleus pulposus.* The bands of the anulus fibrosus fuse with the bone surface at the sides of the vertebrae, but not in front. *The nucleus pulposus is composed of living cells,* fibrous filaments embedded in a gelatinous material containing water and salt. *It is this nucleus that absorbs 75 percent of all the pressure of weight of the structure above it and also dulls the shock waves that travel upward through the spine.* It is the hydrolic properties incorporated in the visco-elastic structure of this ball-shaped nucleus which counteracts the effects of these forces, also by pressing against the vertically oriented fibrous bands that act as elastic springs.

The Disc Has Several Functions

1. It distributes equally, in each direction, the pressure created by weight or load owing to its hydrostatic nucleus. The nucleus has a tremendous ability to absorb water and create a very strong tension within the disc space; this force can reach to twice that of a normal blood pressure. It is this tension that keeps the vertebrae apart and when the joint becomes well-packed, the disc will have the ability to correct force distribution patterns. It is this tension that prevents the articular cartilage of the small facet joints, between the vertebrae on the two sides, to become weight-bearing beyond a certain degree that would be damaging. This damage could begin by the creation of sharp lips; these lips could block the hole through which the nerve passes, thus, one of the causes of pain. A look at Fig. 7 (page 17) will show that the lips of the body of the vertebrae could also become weight-bearing and thus sustain damage.

During the night (horizontal non-weight-bearing posture) the nucleus absorbs a greater amount of water and becomes tense. During the day, when the body is upright, the force of weight will gradually squeeze the water out. This water goes out in the cartilaginous material covering the nucleus; it can go through small holes into the body of the vertebra and join the circulation. It is not only the weight of the upper part of the body that develops a constant pressure on the discs. The muscle groups of the back and front of the vertebral column (Fig. 8, page 20) that maintain the posture of the body have a constant positive tone; this tone in the muscles also brings about a constant pressure on the discs.

Another natural phenomenon which keeps these structures together is the very strong "adhesive" force of vacuum that prevents separation of these otherwise loose structures from the position dictated by the "stays:" muscles and fibrous bands (Figs. 4, page 13, and 8, page 20). The tone and function of these muscles, in conjunction with the fibrous bands and ligaments, dictate a uniform and integrated functional activity, in keeping with the position and curvature of the vertebral column.

Normally, the nucleus absorbs 75 percent of the pressure brought to bear on the disc. The fibrous part of the disc bears only 25 percent of the weight. The nucleus then transfers a part of this pressure to the fibrous rings of the side, which, upon being stretched, keep the nucleus as well as the whole structure of the disc taut and force absorbing all over.

2. Acting as a natural "roller bearing," it allows the vertebrae to move in different directions because the joint has elastic properties.

3. It acts as a buffer to force transmitted up and down the spine in man, and allows coiling and springing out by the quadrupeds.

4. During the normal function of the disc, the facet joints on either side of the spinal processes are kept at a correct distance apart, preventing damage to these joints, as explained above.

5. It maintains a normal size hole or *foramen* for easy and

unhindered passage of the nerve (Fig. 3, page 12).

6. It adds height to the spinal column—about six inches. Its shrinkage between morning and evening (during work) can account for a difference in height of from one and one-half to two centimeters. Taking a close look at Fig. 4, page 13, you will notice there are two thick fibrous bands, or ligaments, stretching in front and at the back of the actual body of the vertebrae.

At the back, the disc and the fibrous band fuse with the lip of the vertebrae above and below, acting as an anchor or stay for the disc, as well as the two connecting vertebrae.

In front, the disc and the ligament fuse together, but they do not fuse with the front lip of the vertebrae. The ligament slides upward and downward and connects, very strongly, to the front of the body of the vertebra away from the lip above and below. This variation in the anatomical attachment of the disc and the vertebrae determines the special functional role of the disc. This type of attachment creates a potential space between the disc and the vertebra in front and not in the back, because in the body, if two distinct tissues do not firmly connect, a potential *anatomical space* will be created between them. Here, I am adopting the anatomical definition exposed by Kapandji's "the physiology of the joints"[28] and not Gray's anatomy.

The Significance of This Hidden Anatomical Space

In the animal kingdom, this anatomical characteristic is very important. Upon watching a dog, a horse, or a deer run, one sees how they coil the body, push with the hind legs, and then stretch in the air, landing on their front legs. This coiling and stretching is the sequence of motion that brings about the actual progress in rapid forward movement.

In the upright man, this coiling and springing has been very finely translated to the walking motion. Man brings one leg forward, leaving the body behind on the other leg, and then throws the weight of the rest of the body onto the forward leg. To have total ability to make the move and change the position of one vertebra in relation to the other, and in order to be able to stretch the joints in sequence for this action to be smooth, the front lips of the vertebrae must be free, and that potential space *must* exist—and that is exactly why it *does* exist. A component of this walking movement is the creation of a momentary vacuum in the anatomical space.

Figure 30 represents the common symbols of the vector of force. Two opposing and in-line forces will distribute evenly. Two opposing and inclined forces will distribute more toward the open angle.

In a movement that coils the vertebrae with force, a strong component of that force will direct itself backwards. And since it is the disc that has to transfer the force, it would undoubtedly travel with the force, if it was free. Since it is

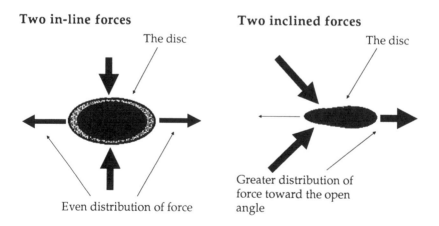

Two in-line forces   **Two inclined forces**

The disc   The disc

Even distribution of force   Greater distribution of
                                  force toward the open
                                  angle

Fig. 30: *Represents vectors of force—showing the distribution of force that will direct the disc to move toward the spinal cord and the nerve after prolonged bad posture and/or loss of the hydrolic pressure of the disc core.*

connected to the front ligament, during the act of stretching the ligament will act like the gut of a bow and draw the disc back as if it were an arrow.

Force of Vacuum Hydrating the Disc

This act of opening the front vertebral space and stretching the firm front ligament covering the gap between the two vertebrae must enhance the force of *vacuum* that exists between the vertebrae. It is this force that keeps these structures together. This force of vacuum, which can be very significant, now brought to the front of the intervertebral space, must also help draw the disc back into position. *This force of vacuum does yet another thing: It must also draw water into the space from the surrounding tissue.*

It must be assumed that if the disc, through the pressure of the "press," has been squeezed of its precious water, this property of local vacuum will facilitate and add to the osmotic process involved in therehydration of the disc. It must be assumed that it is this force of vacuum that maintains the full hydration of the disc tissue (the nucleus pulposus in particular) reestablishing its *full* hydrostatic properties, all these fine adjustments are locked into body movement. It is possible that in some circumstances, if there is a certain amount of dehydration in the area, the force of vacuum may force a *gas separation* and collect gas in the space between the vertebrae.

The shape of the vertebral column was discussed at the beginning of this presentation. It was said that the normal vertebral column has three natural curves; Fig. 1(page 11) was presented in support of this statement. It was said that the column acts as a "coiled spring" to give full support to the head and its brain contents, without allowing the reflection of forces generated during motion to be transmitted to the brain. It was said that the vertebral column and the muscles

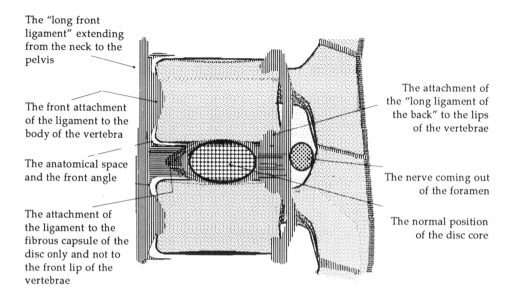

The "long front ligament" extending from the neck to the pelvis

The front attachment of the ligament to the body of the vertebra

The anatomical space and the front angle

The attachment of the ligament to the fibrous capsule of the disc only and not to the front lip of the vertebrae

The attachment of the "long ligament of the back" to the lips of the vertebrae

The nerve coming out of the foramen

The normal position of the disc core

Fig. 31: *Sketch of normal discs with round nucleus pulposis, showing the unobstructed position of the nerve passing through the foramen.*

surrounding the spine act as an integrated unit. That is to say, the muscles give and take all the time to maintain the upright position of the human body, while the fibrous bands and ligaments maintain a firm hold of the bones.

Man, by a gradual turn of the hip joint and the pelvis, has achieved an upright posture at the expense of the discs becoming weight-bearing. The body, under this new situation, has managed to retain a minimal safety margin. By retaining a line of force of gravity that acts to the front of the body, while the back muscles retain an upright posture, the very slightly open space between the vertebrae is maintained in front—in the lumbar region in particular. In other words, the resultant vector of forces direct the pressure to the open angle, as in Fig. 24 (page 42). Therefore, the disc is retained in position.

Should this angle change and, through bad posture, the posterior spaces open up, the line of force will drive the discs and their nuclei backward in the direction of the spinal cord and the nerve roots coming out of the foramina

Here, it should be noted, if an adverse situation arises affecting the integrity of any disc, it will affect more than one disc. It is true that symptoms are highlighted to be from one origin, but postoperative problems, very often seen, demonstrate a more extensive pathology than the one disc operated on.

Figure 31 is a rough sketch of healthy discs, with round and firm nuclei, maintaining the open passageways for the nerves that pass through without obstruction, also to the spinal cord that is positioned in the canal at the back of the discs.

Figure 32 is the same sketch with the open angle facing backward.

The line of force acting on the disc will drive it toward the nerve root and the spinal cord. Depending upon the type and duration of the pressure, the disc may shrink and force the ligament at the back to press on the nerve or the cord to

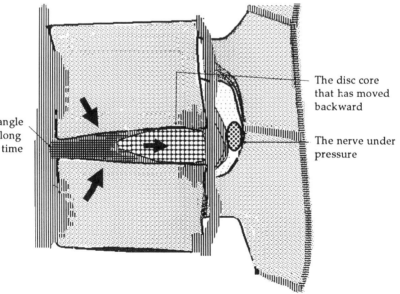

The disc core that has moved backward

The front angle closed for long periods of time

The nerve under pressure

Fig. 32: *Sketch of the disc squeezed backward by closing the front angle of the intervertebral disc spaces for a prolonged period of time, resulting in the pinching of the nerve against the bony part of the foramen.*

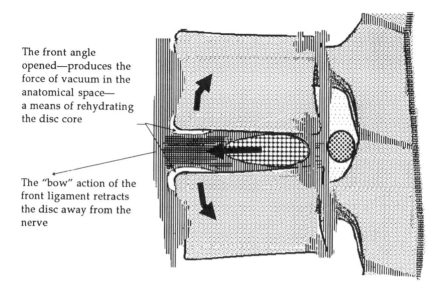

The front angle opened—produces the force of vacuum in the anatomical space—a means of rehydrating the disc core

The "bow" action of the front ligament retracts the disc away from the nerve

Fig. 33: *This sketch is supposed to show the effect of forcing open the front corrective angle, causing a stretching effect on the anterior longitudinal ligament and forcing it to act like the string of a bow, drawing away the disc which is attached to it. At the same time, a vacuum is produced, drawing water into the front space, thus promoting the hydrolic property of the nucleus of the disc. This corrective procedure will affect all the discs that may have been displaced.*

the point of pain or weakness of the muscles in the leg. The disc may, at times, rupture and force the soft nucleus out of its confine, producing the appropriate symptoms.

If the disc is not firm and the nucleus is not absorbing most of the pressure, it is possible that the fibrous ring of the disc may have to bear more of the forces generated. This could involve the "adhesive" properties of vacuum when, with a sudden separation of the upper and lower vertebrae, part of the ring may follow one vertebra and the rest follow the other vertebra, inducing the beginnings of the tear seen after sudden movement of the spine.

Figure 33 is a sketch that demonstrates the corrective effect when the front lip of the intervertebral spaces are opened. All of the intervertebral discs of the region will benefit proportionately from the corrective effect of the front angle of the intervertebral spaces being opened. This sketch is intended to show the effect of the pull by the attachment of the ligament to the front of the discs, as well as the creation of an actual space between the body of the vertebrae and the disc, generating a force of vacuum. This vacuum would assist the disc to slide back to its original position, and would also draw water into the space and encourage the nucleus to hydrate itself much faster than the rate induced by osmotic forces. It is hypothetically possible that this vacuum would encourage a movement of the substance of the nucleus pulposus back to its original position, even if protruded from a rupture. Pain relief is an indication that a retraction of the pulp is a possibility.

The above explanation should clearly give an idea of the conditions that bring about disc problems and the subsequent pathology that follows disc shrinkage. Let us summarize the major points discussed. Firstly, water content within the disc, particularly the nucleus of the disc, establishes the efficiency of the disc as a weight-bearing, force-buffering, joint-packing anatomical organ within the spinal column. Secondly, constant pressure will squeeze the disc substance and reduce its water contents. Thirdly, a uniform, inclined force, brought to bear on the disc, will generate a strong component of that force toward the open angle, encouraging a displacement of the disc. Fourthly, the constant tone of the back muscle group, covering the column, is responsible for maintaining the upright position and open angle of the front part of the intervertebral space, preventing the effect of an uneven pressure on the disc from displacing it. Fifthly, the increase in the gap in front will act as a retractor to the disc, by direct pull of the attachment of the ligament to the disc body and also by creation of a vacuum force; this vacuum not only draws the disc substance, it also draws water into the space, promoting a rehydration of the disc at a faster pace than the osmotic properties of the nucleus would bring about. Finally, this retraction and the rehydration of the disc is absolutely essential to relief from weight pressure on the facet joints at the back of the body of the vertebrae (which, in the long run, may develop bony spurs), as well as releasing pressure from the nerve tissue in the vicinity of the backward driven disc or its nucleus.

Accordingly, if we are to achieve relief from the pain of disc displacement, we have to make sure that our body is optimally hydrated so that water can leave the main circulatory systems and hydrate the disc core. We must also ensure that the front angle of the intervertebral space is kept more open, until corrective restitution to the physical properties and positioning of the disc has taken place. Because the bone marrow and blood-forming cells in the body of vertebrae depend on "free water" for their development and maturation,[1] they will exercise their priority over the disc requirement, if there is a general state of dehydration in the body. When the body is generally dehydrated and at the same time the disc is squeezed of its water content, and this water enters the vertebral bone marrow through the small holes in the flat surfaces of the vertebra that are in contact with the discs above and below, the lost water may not be fully available again for the complete rehydration of the disc's core.

Posturally Induced Retraction and Intermittent Vacuum Reduction of Prolapsed Lumbar Intervertebral Disc

Before any action is taken, a rough diagnosis must be made to determine that the origin of the pain is from the disc, and not from other, more serious disorders. A low back pain that has lasted on and off for some time, eventually developing into a more localized pain, often radiating down the leg, is a fair *indication* that it may be a problem arising from the displacement of one of the intervertebral discs. The word "indication" is used to denote that other conditions can also produce such a picture, but the pathology of the disc and the 5th and 4th lumbar discs in particular is, by far, the most common condition causing such a picture. In any case, the process for the treatment of the disc is not drastic and the result will reveal itself soon enough.

During the time that I have been practicing this method of treatment, I have found a very useful, simple diagnostic sign. Fig. 9 (page 24) reveals, as you will see, that the spinal processes of the vertebrae are almost under the skin of the back, as marked on the skin of the human model shown in the picture. Often, slight pressure of the point of one finger in between the tip of the bony processes and to the side of them (Fig. 9, page 24) will localize the tender and painful disc region.

It is interesting to note that during the process of treatment this tenderness or pain will diminish until it disappears totally, at the same time that the referred pain in the leg gradually draws upward until it is felt no more. It has been my experience that if the condition has not become chronic with progressive local bone pathology and/or after repeated surgery, the exercises with the pillows will normally produce relief after about half an hour. With "first time" apprehension, it may take a short while longer, or even a second try, before the process is understood and carried out efficiently and without anxiety. *It should be appreciated that the human spinal column is capable of extensive forward and backward bending; in this exercise, the required deflection is no more than a small fraction of that capability.*

The Method of Disc Reduction

Four pillows are the only equipment you will need! The pillows must not be too wide, but should be firm, so that by placing one pillow over the other (12 inches) and then the weight of your body on top of them, the two pillows will have a height of about 6 inches. The purpose of these pillows is to temporarily make your body subject to the principles of the force of gravity applicable to horizontal vertebral columns.

You will need to place the two sets of pillows on the floor, about 50 centimeters (or one and one-half feet) apart (Fig. 10, page 25). This distance, of course, depends on your individual height. Kneel on the edge of the front pillows, with your hands on the ground, and *very gently* slide your body forward and lay your chest on the two distant pillows; in this way you will position the area of the pain in your back at exactly equal distance between the two sets of pillows—Fig. 11, pages 26 and 27.

By positioning your body accurately, you will make sure that the greatest opening is brought about in the region of the displaced disc. Because of the spasm of the back muscles, at first your spine will be stiff and unresponsive to the new position—Fig. 11 D (page 27). You should try to relax your back. The best way to relax is to take deep breaths, purposefully timed deep breaths, in such a way that they will produce movement in your spine, forcing it to move up and down.

If need be, this movement should be carried out purposefully until the spine achieves an easy up-and-down mobility.

This up-and-down mobility will keep opening and partially closing the front intervertebral spaces of the entire lumbar region—Fig. 12 (page 28) and Fig. 13 (page 29). In this way, the corrective influences of tendon retraction and vacuum reduction are brought about for *all* of the discs, Fig. 33 (page 84), just like the blacksmith's bellows at the air-drawing phase. In this situation, when the chest also becomes weight-bearing during the deep respiration, the diaphragm and the abdominal muscles take up the responsibility of drawing the air in and forcing it out, thereby creating an additional effect of intermittent vacuum within the abdomen, supplementing the intervertebral vacuum's action on the disc. By now the abdominal muscles should start to relax as the spine begins to move.

This relaxation will bring the abdomen closer to the ground, but not yet touching the ground. If your abdomen touches the ground from the beginning, you should raise the height of the pillows, because the weight of your abdominal mass should force a bend in your back, somewhat like Fig. 14 (page 30).

The same knowledge is applicable to the problems of the discs of the neck and chest region; although one has to improvise for the neck (such as doing the same type of intermittent backward extension of the neck, by resting the forehead on the back of a chair when bending the body downward, or even intermittently bending the head and neck backward), the following process can also help thoracic disc problems.

Having settled into this position and rhythm, in between every few episodes of deep inhalation you should relax so that you do not get dizzy. After a short relaxation, still on the pillows, you should start raising backward first one leg and then the other. This movement should be very slow and purposeful, to a height manageable with comfort, a few times with one leg and then changing to the other. This movement of the legs brings about a slight rotation of the spine, assisting in the movement and correct positioning of the displaced discs. Another effect of this leg-raising from behind is the added enforcement of the spinal movement to open the front angle of the spaces.

After a few periods of deep inhalation and raising of the legs, the abdomen should be relaxed and almost touching the ground, as indicated in Fig. 14 (page 30). This position brings about an exaggerated natural curvature of the lumbar region of the vertebral column.

From the moment the abdomen becomes relaxed to the extent mentioned to the effective reduction of the displacement of the disc, relief of total pain will not be long in coming. These instructions should be carried out until there is no pain when the fingertip presses on the spot that was painful before.

After a few more minutes of relaxed breathing, you should slide sideways on to the floor and remain on the floor for about five minutes to allow the overstretched ligaments and tendons to tighten up before attempting to get up without arching your back. You should first sit up, then get on your knees, followed by slowly rising to your feet.

Essential Points to Observe

For a few days, you should not make any back-bending motions nor carry heavy loads. Any motion requiring a lift of loads off the ground should be made by bending your knees and keeping the back upright, raising the load by straightening your legs rather than bending the back—Fig. 23 B (page 41).

These precautions are necessary to allow the stretched fibrous tissues time to develop strength and tone once again. A series of exercises to strengthen the back muscles is absolutely essential. If you make sure to strengthen the back muscles, and refrain from adopting a posture that opens the back side of the intervertebral spaces, forcing the disc out of position once again, you will manage to keep the disc in its correct position and remain pain-free.

The harmful postures stated in the previous section should be strictly avoided. With repeated adoption of the above proposed corrective postures, improvement in very chronic cases has also been seen.

The Exercises to Strengthen Your Back Muscles

The exercises, by and large, are a repeat of the procedures used for the reduction of the displaced disc. If you sweat with exercise, you should drink water in anticipation of body water loss. In this way you will prevent dehydration and hemoconcentration (making blood concentrated by the loss of its water). All of the problems of the body, including the manufacture and deposit of cholesterol at the arterial walls, begin with the initial steps that produce hemoconcentration. This recommendation also applies to sauna and steam bath "addicts," who try to keep the weighing scale happy at the expense of dehydrating the body. *It has been shown that with increase in age it takes much longer to rehydrate the body to the same level as before when forced dehydration has been induced.*[25]

The basic exercises demonstrated in the preceding section are devised to strengthen the spinal muscles. As a result of improving the local circulation, the efficiency and the co-ordination of the tendon reflexes will improve, and the fibrous bands, tendons, and ligaments will also get stronger. At some later stage, you may want to use leg weights to increase the exercise value of your muscle contractions.

Back Pain and Body Position

In this book, I have explained a physiological and postural approach to back pain. On the face of it, my explanation might seem to contradict the current understanding when professional advice recommends a posture with legs drawn in and pillows placed under the knees when sleeping on one's back or in a fetal position. Often, the back pain seems to subside after a few days of rest in these positions (with the help of some pain-killers). This postural effect has a simple explanation that may interest you.

When upright, the human body leans forward all the time, and the back muscles keep pulling the body backward all the time. This cause-and-effect response of the body is automatic and constant. Under a constant central nervous system directive, the back muscles maintain this posture. The only time these muscles relax is, when lying down, the opposing front muscles are told to pull the body forward, when the back muscles can then partially relax by a release from the central nervous system command to remain fully in tone (when standing, the burden on the back muscles is increased). When lying on one's back and bending the knees, the back muscles are released from any constantly operative central nervous contraction command (muscle tone that eventually causes spasm). This simple bed rest approach to back pain is palliative; it does not affect the very basic body dehydration reason for the back pain.

What I have exposed is the root of the problem and how to correct it; also, by maintaining a "stronger" and a more efficient physiology of the muscles of the back, how to prevent future back pain.

Essential Precautions

These special floor exercises should be carried out often and with an increase in intensity and duration of the effort.

Before we finish this short manual, let us touch on the importance of the quantity of your water intake as an absolutely essential first step of this treatment procedure. The thirst sensation is not a reliable indicator for water intake; you can be dehydrated and yet not feel thirsty. If the cells of the body are generally or locally dehydrated and fluids of the body more concentrated than they should be, they will not release their own essential commodity to the matrix of the nucleus pulposus to build up its volume and those hydrolic properties that jack up one vertebra from the other. The whole problem of disc degeneration starts from this very simple step in the not fully water-compensated physiology of the body. *Everyone* needs at least one and one-half to two liters of water (three pints) every day of his/her life, thirsty or not. *Coffee, tea, and alcohol, although fluids containing water, do not serve as water for the cells; they are dehydrating agents.*

Final Recommendations

Having read this self-treatment book, you should now have a basic understanding about the physiology and function of your intervertebral discs, particularly the 5th lumbar disc—Fig. 27, page 46.

There may come a time when you will become impatient with your disc problems and think you should do something about them. Make it a principle to consult more than one person; there are too many knife-happy "experts." Surgical operations are not always the answer to your problem; indeed, *they may add to it*. If you read any self-respecting book on the subject, you will see that they have the same opinion; they always recommend conservative treatment as a first "must" in this condition.

Recently, a new injection procedure has emerged as a "conservative" step in the treatment of disc problems. Chymopapain is an extract of the papaya tree. Injection of this material in the disc is said to dissolve some of the substances in the problematic disc. Although now in vogue, the rationale about this method of treatment is being questioned.

An editorial article in *The Lancet* (a very respected medical journal) has addressed this very subject. It seems that the activity of this chemical is limited to only four percent of the composition of the disc, hardly a significant effect. The highlight of this article is the discussion around the comparison of this substance with a placebo. It seems that a placebo has as good an effect as chymopapain in relieving pain. (A placebo is an inert substance used for comparison with the drug under investigation.) The discussion is interesting, but one statement made is *very* important: "Thus, whilst chymopapain is clearly shown to be superior to saline in double-blind studies, there is no evidence that it is better than nothing—i.e., leaving the disc derangement entirely to its own devices." This seems to be very sound advice to those facing this problem at its early stages of development. A conservative attitude to this problem is the height of prudence. The first steps in that direction are regular fluid intake and appropriate exercises to strengthen the *back* muscles to keep your spine upright and well-adjusted to the needs of your body.

Some may want to go to chiropractitioners for manipulation of spine. The basic information and the recommended exercises contained in this booklet may serve as the initial step in that direction and you might succeed in being your own chiropractor.

Until a more complete understanding is brought to attention, the reader is advised to think of the body as if it were a satellite in space. In the same way that space dwellers will have taken an environment compatible to their physiological survival in space, man should be looked at as if he were a "space station" of water-dwellers. Water-dwellers bring their system of economy and power structure with them, a system that only understands survival in a water medium because, within the "space station," all transports are water carried, even within the cells that seem to have microstream systems that carry the components of manufacturing systems to and from the assembly lines. This we call DNA complex (the scientific reader with an enquiring mind could find information about this idea in the articles by Dieter Weiss, *et al*. No. 20 in the Bibliography).

Another important phenomenon about water around and inside the cell emerges from the way the water-dwelling cells have evolved an energy-generating system very similar to hydroelectric power generation. If we dam water and create a "waterhead," the force of which is used to run generators in a power plant and provide electrical energy, the cells use the difference in water content of the cells and the water content of the solution outside the cells and, by exposing the cell's many generators (the cation pumps) to this "waterhead" outside, the cells generate electrical potential that is stored in the cells' chemical batteries (adenosine triphosphate, ATP), subsequently to be used for units of work needed for cell survival.

Bibliography

1. Cicoria, A.D. and Hempling, H.G;

a) Osmotic Properties of a Proliferating and Differentiating Line of Cells from the Bone Marrow of the Rat; pp. 105,127;

b) Osmotic Properties of Differentiating Bone Marrow Precursor Cells: Membrane Permeability to Non-Electrolytes; pp. 129-136; The Journal of Cellular Physiology, Vol 105; Febuary 1980.

2. Batmanghilidj, F.; Peptic Ulcer Disease; A Natural Method for Prevention and Treatment; The Journal of the Iranian Medical Council, Vol. 6, No. 4, pp. 280-282, September 1982.

3. Batmanghelidj, F.; A New and Natural Method of Treatment of Peptic Ulcer Disease, J. Clin. Gastroenterology, 5: 203-205, 1983.

4. Batmanghelidj, F.; Revolution of Water in Medical Treatments, pp. 1-199 (in Persian language) Rowim, 1985-6

5. Batmanghelidj, F.; "Vacuum Treatment" of Low Back and Sciatic Pain, pp. 199-251, Revolution of Water in Medical Treatments; (in Persian language) Rowim Co., 1985-6 ISBN 0-934497-72-9.

6. Batmanghelidj, F.; Pain; A Need for Paradigm Change, Anticancer Research, Vol. 7, No. 5B, pp. 971-990 Sept-Oct 1987.

7. Batmanghelidj, F.; Can Functions of Histamine in the Body Offer Explanation for Some of the Problems Seen in Gastroenterology?, Sci Med Simplified (to be published1991).

8. Batmanghelidj, F.; Is Cell Membrane Receptor Protein Down-Regulation also a Hydrodynamic Phenomenon?, Sci Med Simplified (to be published1991).

9. Batmanghelidj, F.; Neurotransmitter Histamine: an Alternate Viewpoint; 3rd Interscience World Conference on Inflammation, Antirheumatics, Analgesics, Immunomodulators; Book of Abstracts page 37 (A137), Monte Carlo 15-18-March 1989; Also, Sci Med Simplified (the full article - a Foundation for the Simple in Medicine publication). Vol. I, pp. 7-39. April 1990.

10. West, IC.; The Biochemistry of Membrane Transports, Chapmen and Hall.

11. Wiggin, Philippa M.; A Mechanism of ATP-Driven Cation Pumps. pp266-269 Biophysics of Water, Eds. Felix Frank and Shiela F. Mathias, John Wiley and Sons LTD. 1982.

12. Hempling, H.G.; Osmosis: The Push and Pull of Life; pp. 205-214, Biophysics of Water, Eds. Felix Frank and Shiela F. Mathias, John Wiley and Sons LTD. 1982.

13. Hayden D. A.; Water, Permeation Through Lipid Bilayer Membranes: pp. 269-271, Biophysics of Water, Eds. Felix Frank and Shiela F. Mathias, John Wiley and Sons LTD. 1982.

14. Selvaggio, A.M.; Schwatz, J.H.: Bengele, H.H. and Alexander, E.A.; Kinetics of the Na+-H+ Antiporter as Assessed by the Change in Intracellular PH in MDCK Cells; pp. C553-C562, The American Physiological Society, 0363-6143, 1986.

15. Livne A.; Veitch, R.; Grinstein, S.; Balfe, J.W.; Marquez-Julio, A.; and Rothstein, A.; Increased Platelet Na+-H+ Exchange Rates in Essential Hypertension: Application of a Novel Test; pp. 533-536, Lancet March 7, 1987.

16. Eisen V.; Munday, M.R. and Slater, J.D.H.; Role of Kinninase II in the Regulation of Renin Secretion; KininIV, Part A, Eds. Lowell M. Greenbaum and Harry S. Matrgolius, Plenum Press, 1986.

17. Beierwalter, W.H.G. and Carretero, O.A.; Kallikrein and Kinins Independently Stimulate Release From Isolated Rat Glomeruli; pp. 265-272, Kinin IV, Part A, Eds. Lowell M. Greenbaum and Harry S. Margolius, Plenum Press, 1986.

18. Seto, S.; Rabit, S.F.; Maitra, S.R.; Wu, N.J; Effect of Sodium Restriction and Corticosteroids on Glandular Kallikrein in Plasma and Submanibular Glands; Plenum Press, 1986.

19. Douglas, W.W; Polypetides-Angiotensin Plasma Kinins, and Others; pp.647-667, Goodman and Gilman's the Pharmacological Basis of Therapeutics, MacMillan 1980.

20. Weiss, Dieter G. and Guenter W. Gross; Intracellular Transport in Nerve Cell Processes: The Chromatorgraphic Dynamics of Axoplasmic Transport; pp. 387-396, Biological Structures and Coupled Flows, Edited by A. Oplatka and M. Balaban, Academic Press, 1983.

21. Makara, Gabor B.: Mechanism by Which Stressful Stimuli Activate the Pituitary-Adrenal System, pp. 149-153, Federation Proceeding Vol 44, No.1, Pt.2 January 1985.

22. Fitzsimon, J.T.; Mechanism of Thirst and Sodium Appetite in Hypovolaemia; pp. 385-402, Recent Advances in Physiology, Ed. P.F. Baker, Churchill Livingstone, 1984.

23. Thirst and Osmoregulation in the Elderly, Editorial: pp. 1017-1018, Lancet, November 3, 1984.

24. Streen, B.; Lundgren, B.K.; Isaksson, B.; Body Water in the Elderly; p.101, Lancet, Jan.12, 1985.

25. Phillips, P.A.; Rolls, B.J.; Ledingham, J.G.C.; Mary L. Forsling; James. J. Morton Morgan J. Crowe, and Leopold Wollner; Reduced Thirst After Deprivation in Healthy Elderly Men, New England Journal of Medicine, pp. 753-759, 1984.

26. Bruce, A.; Anderson, M.; Arvidsson, B. and Isaksson, B.; Body Water Composition. Prediction of Normal Body Potassium, Body Water Body Fat in Adults on the Basis of Body Height, Body Weight and Age: Scand,. J. Clin. Lab. Invest. 40-461-473, 1980.

27. Pain; Meaning and Management; Eds. W. Lynn Smith, Harold Merskey and Steven Gross. Sp Medical and Scientific Books, 1980.

28. The Physiology of the Joints; I.A. Kapandji, Vol. 3 Churchill Livingstone. 1974.

29. The Slipped Disc; James Cyriax, Gower 1970-5-1980.

30. Clinics in Sports Medicine; Vol. 6/November 2 April 1987, Overuse Injuries, Ed. Letha Y. Hunter-Griffin, W.B. Saunders & Co., 1987.

31. Wood, George W.; Lower Back Pain and Disorders of Intervertebral Disc, pp. 3255-3321, Campbell's Operative Orthopaedics, Ed. A.H. Crenshaw. 1987.

32. The Back; pp. 1483-1519, Orthopaedics Principles and Their Application. Ed. Samuel L. Turek. Lippincott Co. 1984.

33. Intervertebral Disc Injuries; Chapter 31 pp. 620 and 629-631; The Spine; A Radiological Text and Atlas, Ed. Bernard S. Eptein, Fourth Edition 1976.

34. Raines, Richard J.; Intervertebral Disc Fissures (Vacuum Intervertebral Disc); pp. 964-966, December 1953, American Journal of Roentgenology Radium Therapy and Nuclear Medicine,

35. Mark, James T.; Gas in Intervertebral Disc, pp.804-809 November, 1953, American Journal of Roentgenology Radium Therapy and Nuclear Medicine, 1953.

36. Chymopapain and the Intervertebral Disc; The Lancet, pp. 843-845, October 11, 1986.

37. Thoracic and Lumbar Spines; pp. 17-29, Common Vertebral Joint Problems, Gregory P. Grieve, Churchill Livingstone, 1981.

38. Katchalski-Katzir, E.; Conformational Change in Macromolecules; Biorheology, 21, pp. 57-74, 1984.